The Yogic Lifestyle

A Foundation for Freedom

Melissa K Lavery

Table of Contents

Introduction

Freedom.

What does that look like to you? To many, it is the ability to exist without restriction, to live your life on your own terms. In the United States, freedom is built into the bedrock. It is the underlying pulse that drives and protects its people. But according to yoga, birthed in India, freedom takes on a different form. Freedom is enlightenment. It is removing all obstacles to unlocking the ultimate truth: Everything is one divine and eternal consciousness. Yoga is the path to actualization.

In Sanskrit, a beautiful and sacred language you will see throughout these pages, the word yoga translates to "union". Union, in this sense, is the ultimate liberation from suffering. It is the joy of Being. It is the contentment felt when one sheds all earthly desires, attachments, and fears. It is unfettered freedom. The East (India) and the West (the U.S.) are vastly different in their cultures and histories, and yet, the people of the West have been adopting and assimilating yoga into their lives for over a century. But, as expected, its practice is unique to the American concept.

Yoga is more than a result, it is a journey, and it is through this journey that one can find real freedom. The point of this book is to help people live a more yogic lifestyle in a contemporary society, whether people are looking to improve their personal yoga practice or to incorporate the benefits more easily into everyday life, which is what a yoga practice is: a way to live.

The words in this book are primarily based on the wisdom of "The Yoga Sūtras of Patañjali," a compilation of "threads" (*sūtras*) that put into words all that is yoga. The source material for most of this book comes from this text, translated by Śrī Svāmī Saccidānanda.

Although many forms of yoga exist, "The Yogic Lifestyle: A Foundation for Freedom" is based on the teachings of *Aṣṭāṅga Yoga* and the eight-limbed path to achieve ultimate liberation. But instead of displaying this information in order of those limbs, I have chosen a different path, one that can be easily understood from the circumstances that surround us in a contemporary and Western society. A person does not need to be a yoga practitioner or have any experience with yoga to gain wisdom from the *Yoga Sūtras*.

This book focuses on relationships first (ultimate union) as a guide to moral integrity and purity. Next is health, as one needs a sound body, mind, and spirit to achieve union. And third, the text focuses on abundance, not necessarily in gaining vast amounts of riches, but the kind of prosperity that allows us to actualize financial freedom and supportive resources. It is through a yogic lifestyle that one can actualize liberation, changing the world from the inside out.

As stated earlier, the intention of this book is to bring the ancient and often foreign aspects of yoga to anyone who is looking to begin or enhance their practice. Sanskrit is just as much a part of yoga as English is to Shakespeare: Its use is paramount to understanding the nuance, the spirit behind the word.

The use of Sanskrit in this book is presented from the main source material, found in "The Yoga Sūtras of Patāñjali", translated by Śrī Svāmī Saccidānanda. The use of accent marks and definitions (except for yoga poses) are directly from this source. You will notice that in some places, a term will be capitalized, while in another place, it is not:

• Limbs of *Aṣṭāṅga Yoga* will be capitalized when referring directly to the limb (like a level or main concept); they will remain in lower case when referred to as their definition or action.

• The term yoga is not capitalized or italicized, because it is well known among Western society. However, it is worth mentioning that it is still Sanskrit. In addition, any specific type of yoga or *āsana* postures will be both capitalized and italicized.

• The term *sūtra* is capitalized when referring to a specific *sūtra* (thread). The *Yoga Sūtras* refer to "The Yoga Sūtras of Patāñjali".

• A note about *Samādhi*. According to many style guides, *Samādhi* remains capitalized throughout, regardless of its reference. The reason for this distinction is that *Samādhi* is a proper noun, a place—a state of being—as well as a limb of *Aṣṭāṅga Yoga*.

I

The Yogic Lifestyle: A Foundation for Relationships

1

Yama: How to Eliminate Suffering and Cultivate a Better Relationship with the World

"Yama consists of nonviolence, truthfulness, non-stealing, continence, and non-greed."
-The Yoga Sūtra of Patāñjali, 2.30

The Golden Rule transcends time and culture. Like the precious metal, this sage advice can transmute the lead in our external experiences to refined and joyous living. Treating others the way you wish to be treated seems simple, but with the complexities that exist in the world, we often find ourselves struggling with interpersonal relationships. However, with the ancient wisdom of yoga, it is possible to travel the path of limited suffering and abide in a better relationship with the outside world.

Our relationship with the world is multifaceted: We exist in communion with family, friends, lovers, coworkers, neighbors, and even strangers. Every day we experience life alongside other beings, which include animals and our environment. These relationships span from within the walls of our homes to the vast reaches of the planet. The beliefs, practices, and behaviors we espouse can differ greatly from any one of these entities.

To practice yoga and live a yogic lifestyle, one must follow the eight-fold path described in the *Yoga Sūtras*. As described many times throughout this book, the path consists of the following eight limbs:

- *Yama* (abstinences)

- *Niyama* (observances)

- *Āsana* (postures)

- *Prāṇāyāma* (breath control)

- *Pratyāhāra* (sensory withdrawal)

- *Dharāṇā* (concentration)

- *Dyhāna* (meditation)

- *Samādhi* (absorption)

This chapter will focus on the first limb or rung of this ladder—*Yama*. In Sanskrit, *yama* translates to "moral discipline". This discipline describes the thoughts, speech, and actions we put out into the external world. There are five *yamas* we must consider when relating to the world, which are reflected in many spiritual practices and governmental laws:

- *Ahiṁsā* (non-violence)

- *Satya* (truthfulness)

- *Asteya* (non-stealing)

- *Brahmacharya* (continence)

- *Aparigrahā* (non-covetousness)

When we abide by these ethical principles, laid out in many teachings, including the *Yoga Sūtras*, we can make a positive impact on everything we encounter and work to eliminate suffering on a collective level.

How to Control Your Behavior to Support External Relationships

Yoga practice and application is about strengthening your physical, mental, and emotional capacities. The intention of living a yogic lifestyle is to improve your life, relieve suffering, and obtain peace. A part of this peace includes how you interact with the world around you and how the world reacts to your action (or inaction).

Karma is our actions, words, and thoughts that elicit a response. This response is an energetic impression, the low- or high-level energies of our emotions—sadness/joy, love/hate, fear/courage, etc. According to Nicolai Bachman, author of "The Path of the Yoga Sutras", *karma* can come from us or can come from an external source, such as a conversation, movie, or other sensory experience.

Whether these impressions are subtle or dramatic, these energies affect our heart-mind. Even the laws of physics acknowledge there exists "an equal and opposite reaction" to an initial action. Think of these actions as ripples in a pond: Eventually, they will move an object downstream.

The impact, imprint, or impression these actions make ultimately become our *saṁskāras*, which means "formations". These mental impressions occur when we intake sensory stimuli and assimilate the experience into our memories. These memories of the event influence our behaviors, whether the event was benign or traumatic.

Every person you meet experiences this phenomenon. Animals, plants, and even the weather/climate demonstrate the repercussions of cause and effect. When we begin to realize the enormous impact each and every action has upon the faculties of our heart-mind, you will understand the importance of emitting positive, high-level energy into the world.

Ahiṁsā (Non-Violence)

"In the presence of one firmly established in nonviolence, all hostilities cease."
-*The Yoga Sūtra of Patāñjali, 2.35*

The first *yama*, or abstinence, is *ahiṁsā*. *Ahiṁsā* is the act of non-violence. Non-violence includes the tenets of compassion, forgiveness, and non-judgement. To practice *ahiṁsā* is to live in a manner that intends to reduce harm in all actions. In a way, all the *yamas* espouse the moral principle that is non-violence. When we abstain from violence, deceit, stealing, misusing our energy, and greed, we work to prevent harm.

The Effects of Violence on Others and Yourself

Violence can include mental, emotional, and physical abuse. When we harm someone, the effects are far reaching. The negative action will influence the person, animal, or object that receives the harmful action. The effects could be that a person or animal retaliates, or becomes deflated and unable to live according to their purpose. An inanimate object can break, which also diminishes its usefulness. We harm others and ourselves in the following ways:

- When we physically hurt a person, animal, nature, or inanimate object, we can cause irreparable damage. We can also suffer through the ramifications of such an event.

- When we think or speak negatively about someone or something, we act to end that person's or object's life. In the same way that physical violence can lead to death or trauma, being cut off from society (through the use of rumors or a bad reputation) is a form of death.

- When we listen to hateful speech, watch violent movies, or participate in activities that emit low-energetic frequencies (fear, anger, ignorance, etc.), we increase our chances of hostility.

- When we react to negativity through retaliatory behaviors, we subject ourselves and others to cycles of violence.

Violence is harmful, because it is disruptive. Adversely, unconditional love and kindness maintain stability. Kindness negates hostility. Hostility begets violence. These behaviors will become cyclical patterns, creating habits that continue to injure all parties involved. The key, according to the *Yoga Sūtras*, is to become the "antidote to violence" (Bachman, p. 146).

How to Practice Nonviolence

To begin acting in a nonviolent and compassionate way, it is essential to see the importance of everything we encounter, treating all objects—alive or inanimate—as purposeful and sacred in their origins.

- Instead squashing unwanted vermin or insects in your home, see each as having a purpose. Try to collect these critters and release them, or let them be.

- Think of someone toward whom you feel hostility or negativity. Intentionally send them good energy, whether love, forgiveness, or understanding.

- Practice the pause. Instead of reacting to negativity with more negativity, take a breath before responding. In your response, make sure to act, speak, and think in a way that imposes minimal damage.

- Consider the ways that violence and low-level energy enter your life. Are you an active participant? Is there a way that you can limit your interaction with these sensory stimuli?

- Pay attention to the ways in which you condone violent actions though your inaction. Try to use your gifts and talents to provide an antidote to the violence of this world.

Satya (Truthfulness)

"To one established in truthfulness, actions and their results become subservient."
-The Yoga Sūtra of Patāñjali, 2.36

Absolute honesty is the focus of the second *yama*. In Sanskrit, *satya* means "truth," and it encompasses thoughts, speech, and actions. For many, telling the truth seems easy, but to practice *satya*, one must not merely tell the truth, but dishonesty must be completely eliminated from everyday life. To live according to this *Sūtra*, a person must apply truthfulness in all areas of his or her life, using the light of faithfulness to create a pure heart-mind.

The Effects of Dishonesty on Others and Yourself

If you wish to practice *ahiṁsā*, *satya* will come naturally. It is impossible to withhold the truth or even produce a white lie if you wish to practice *ahiṁsā*. *Satya* is about pure interactions with others, acting intentionally. If you are unclear at all with your words or actions, then you diminish your trustworthiness. For example, you can tell people that you intend to live a certain way (and even believe these words yourself), but if you do not live out your truth, then your delusions will become a warning to those around you: You are not trustworthy.

- When you pay someone a compliment that is insincere.

- If a friend asks you what you think about something (their outfit, new love interest, or if you are upset with them), it is irresponsible to lie.

- When you make assumptions, use deception, or pass along rumors.

How to Practice Truthfulness

- Always tell the truth, being mindful of limiting harm. You do not need to be rude or accusatory, but it is appropriate to tell people what you prefer, so they understand your sincere desires. This honesty will also limit resentment toward other people's actions or choices.

- Strive to be reliable, matching your actions with your words.

- Refuse to spread misinformation. Do not partake in gossip or attaching your preconceived beliefs to events. Use a clear mind to see events as they occurred and question your own biases.

Asteya (Non-Stealing)

"To one established in non-stealing, all wealth comes."
-The Yoga Sūtra of Patāñjali, 2.37

Asteya encompasses non-stealing in any form: physically taking items, misusing time and materials, depleting your own energy by giving too much, etc. When we take something from someone, whether it be their possessions, peace, or time, we are stealing. We can steal from nature, cultures, other people, employers, and ourselves. Receiving a gift is not considered stealing; however, taking something for granted—which may deplete an energy source—without a grateful attitude or reciprocity, is considered theft.

The Effects of Stealing on Others and Yourself

Linked with *ahiṁsā* and *satya*, *asteya* requires honesty and working to limit harm. There are many ways in which we steal, without realizing the effects on their sources:

- When we throw away, hoard, or misuse goods that can be used by others.

- When we interrupt conversations or ignore people.

- When we take resources from nature without gratitude or replenishing its gifts.

- When we receive the benefit of a mistake and do not rectify the situation.

- When we take an object for our own that belongs to someone else.

- When we plagiarize or use intellectual material, taking credit for its creation.

- When we do not use our time at work appropriately yet receive a paycheck.

Stealing hurts all parties involved. It hurts the person who loses the property, because they can no longer use the property. It can break trust between parties, creating suspicion and fear. Taking time from an employer can limit that source's productivity, and the effects can ripple out on a global scale. Claiming someone's work as our own diminishes the originator's compensation, of which they may need to survive. Hoarding property, food, and money can hurt those who need these resources more than we do. And finally, stealing can hurt the thief because the thief can go to jail, acquire a record, and lose credibility. Work ethic diminishes, resources are not recuperated, and the thief learns nothing about the proper exchange of energy.

How to Practice Non-Stealing

- Pay nature back for oxygen, water, and other natural resources by planting trees, cleaning up the earth, and only taking what is needed.

- When you are privy to a mistake, use honesty to correct it.

- Donate excess money and items that you no longer need.

- Be diligent at work and when claiming what is your creative property.

- Do not interrupt others or waste their time. Be considerate of other people's property.

Brahmacarya (Conservation of Vital Energy)

"By one established in continence, vigor is gained."
-The Yoga Sūtra of Patañjali, 2.38

Brahmacarya is similar to non-stealing, however, the theft is against yourself. When we give of our vital energy, without replenishment, we deplete our physical, mental, and spiritual/emotional stores. This *Sūtra* is about the principle of stamina and controlling our sensory impulses. To practice yoga, one must move away from concern over sensory pleasures and move toward (*carya*) supreme truth (*Brahma*). The sensations of the body deplete the energy we need to reach union within. Although this *Sūtra* is concerned more with the practitioner, the effects of wasting vital energy can harm others, as well.

The Effects of Depleting Vital Energy on Others and Yourself

This *Sūtra* focuses mostly on the physical and emotional aspects of sexual relationships. It is not concerned with strict celibacy, although for some, this is an important aspect of the yogic path. However, it is important to note that this *Sūtra* mostly discusses sexual energy exchange and how inappropriate use of our vital sexual energy can diminish our own health:

- When we consider love only a physical act, we can overindulge in sexual activity. This behavior can cause physical harm to our bodies, and our partners', through sexually transmitted diseases or unwanted pregnancies.

- When we overindulge in any activity in which we give of ourselves, we can experience physical, mental, and emotional fatigue.

- When we equate love with sex, we diminish the holy quality of our bodies.

Conserved vital energy is converted to our subtle body, which is *ojas* or "vigor". Over time, *ojas* creates *tejas*, which is our personal "illumination" and external effects we have on the world.

How to Practice Conservation of Vital Energy

- Practice moderation and control the impulses for appropriate use of vital energy (do not overly give of yourself).

- Be judicious with whom and how you demonstrate physical love.

- Use your vital energy appropriately for physical, mental, and emotional/spiritual stamina.

Aparigrahā (Non-Hoarding)

"When non-greed is confirmed, a thorough illumination of the how and why of one's birth comes."
-The Yoga Sūtra of Patāñjali, 2.39

Aparigrahā is like *asteya*. It is about an intense desire for material goods. *Asteya* focuses more on theft and misuse, while *aparigrahā* focuses on possessiveness, as well as an insatiable desire to consume and hoard material goods.

The Effects of Hoarding on Others and Yourself

When we become preoccupied with possessions, we become slaves to the ego and bound to our earthly attachments:

- When we feel obligated to others as a response to their giving

- When we are more concerned with recognition than progress

- When we act out of the need for power and control, not allowing others to be themselves or have their own opinions

- When we dominate conversations or insult others' opinions

Hoarding power and possessions can harm others and yourself. We lose valuable insight from others when we control the narrative. We feel beholden to others when we do not allow others to give freely, without expectation. And we continue to deplete our vital energy when we cling to earthly attachments, instead of realizing that these materials are temporary and cause static in our relationships.

How to Practice Non-Hoarding

- Eliminate your desire for external possessions so you can focus on your internal status.

- Think of gifts as gifts, not as place markers for obligations later to be paid.

- Allow others to state their points of view. This behavior is especially important for people in places of leadership.

- Manage your desire to participate in consumerism. Purchase only what you need and be an example to others by demonstrating moderation.

Often, it seems as if we are battling the world, with the need to protect ourselves from foreign invaders of our physical space and inner peace. But our relationship with the world is within our control. By choosing to follow the path of yoga and the wisdom of the *Yoga Sūtras*, we can manage our energetic footprint. Our behavior, like everything else, ripples out into the world. Our actions cause reactions. This concept can be explained by the principles of science or spiritual belief—the laws of physics or *karma*. Suffering exists when we tread outside the lines of a pure heart-mind. Through these *sūtras*, you can clean your heart-mind and use its light as a laser beam to enhance your impact on the world.

2

Niyama: How to Cultivate a Better Relationship with Yourself and Commit to Personal Self-Care

"Niyama consists of purity, contentment, accepting but not causing pain, study of spiritual books, and worship of God [self-surrender]."
-The Yoga Sūtra of Patāñjali, 2.32

The measure of happiness is contentment and circumventing that which makes us suffer. Most people seek outside of themselves for happiness. They count their blessings in monetary and material terms: car, house, spouse, body, clothing, and possessions. They use the guidance of consumerism and celebrity to determine what it is that will make them happy.

According to the practice of yoga, happiness is not obtained through monetary wealth or physical beauty. Happiness is achieved when we abide by certain principles that make us pure, strong, and cohesive—inside and out. Yoga means "union". It is through living a yogic lifestyle that one finds union within, not without, and through this union, one can find bliss (*Samādhi*).

The last chapter's focus was on the first of the eight limbs of *Aṣṭāṅga Yoga*, *Yama* (or abstinences), and how they are necessary to live in harmony with the world, its people, animals, and with nature. For this chapter, the focus will be on the second limb, which describes *Niyama*. In Sanskrit, *niyama* is an "observance". These observances lead the practitioner down a path of personal self-care:

- *Śauca* (cleanliness)

- *Saṁtoṣa* (contentment)

- *Tapas* (practice causing positive change)

- *Svādhyāya* (independent study)

- *Īśvara-Praṇidhāna* (humility and faith)

When combined with the *yamas*, these observances and abstinences are akin to that of several religious and spiritual ethical guidelines (the Ten Commandments of Christianity and Judaism, the ten virtues of Buddhism, etc.). These principles will help you to cultivate a positive relationship with yourself, purifying and strengthening your body, mind, and spirit.

How to Cultivate and Support Your Internal Relationship

Practicing *Niyama* is all about personal self-care. If yoga means "union", then the *niyamas* are a series of lampposts on the path toward inner enlightenment. Nothing outside of yourself can bring you bliss, only your attitude, perspective, and inner wisdom can bring you joy. This union refers to meeting yourself, your Source, and connecting with the ever-present Awareness that exists in everything.

Niyama means "observance". As Nicolai Bahman points out, these are like "Internal *yama-s*". We already know that what energy you emit outward comes back to you through your actions (*karma*). The external world will respond to your actions in kind, either creating ease or dis-ease in your life. In the same way, when you begin to make observations about your behavior and its effects on your personal growth and health, you will begin to plan for transformation. This change may be difficult, but it will lead to a place of peace and fulfillment.

The first two *niyamas* are the bridge between your inner and outer worlds. They consist of preparing and maintaining your physical body, as well as living in acceptance of what *is*.

Śauca (Cleanliness)

> *"By purification arises disgust for one's own body and for contact with other bodies."*
> -The Yoga Sūtra of Patāñjali, 2.40

The first *niyama*, or observance, is about purifying the body. Not only does this practice encompass the physical body, but it also refers to keeping a clear heart-mind. In the above *Sūtra*, Śrī Svāmī Saccidānanda translates Patāñjali's words in a way that may make you wince. How is becoming disgusted with one's own body healthy, and how can it lead to contentment?

These words are not intended to make you hate your body; however, they are intended for you to realize and understand that your body (and others') is always impure. And it is in this realization that you come to terms with the fact that your body is temporary and needs consistent care.

Purifying the body includes your mental and emotional energy centers. Cleanliness refers to the following aspects of living:

- Diet and exercise

- Daily hygiene routines

- Being honest and purging your emotions

- Abstaining from substance abuse

- Avoiding behaviors that defile or degrade the body

Living within this cleanliness requires balance. It is not appropriate to be so clean that you live in a state of anxiety and controlling behaviors. Remember, the need to control is an ego-driven behavior. Once we move onto the second *niyama*, the emphasis is on acceptance and contentment.

This *Sūtra* also explains the necessity to limit your physical desire for another's body. This is not to say that sexual contact is unhealthy, because a healthy sex life is important; however, this *Sūtra* means that the lust for another's physical body will bring you less happiness than spiritual union within yourself. Yoga calls the practitioner to support the meeting of both feminine and masculine energies, which reside in all of us. We can do this by balancing our personalities and actions, being both assertive and nurturing. Here, we must observe our imbalances and work to purify the parts of us that are out of balance.

When you practice cleanliness, you work to prepare your body and mind for union. *Śauca* leads to happiness and controlling the senses, which ultimately lead to the necessary changes in one's Self. It is like a meditative practice: When one notices or observes an impure thought, word, or action, then the practitioner can go back to the practices of cleanliness and the process will become more automatic.

How to Practice Cleanliness

The first part of cleanliness is to purify the body. Intertwined are mental and spiritual practices that help to support the mind and emotions. Participating in a daily routine (*dinacharyā*) that puts physical hygiene at the top of your personal care list is essential. An *Āyurvedic* self-care regimen is a good place to start (see the supplement at the end of this book for more information about *Āyurveda*, the sister science of yoga):

1. Begin the day with a prayer or moment of gratitude.

2. Move onto elimination: Go to the bathroom, then cleanse your mouth and body from the night's accumulation of bacteria.

- Scrape the tongue (using a spoon or tongue scraper)

- Gargle with warm saltwater

- Oil swish with sesame oil for 5-20 minutes

- Brush teeth

- Drink a cup of warm (lemon) water.

- Bathe. Wash face and eyes.

3. Move onto strengthening the body through *āsana* (yoga postures).

- A round (three sets) of *Sūrya Namaskār* (Sun Salutations) and/or *Candra Namaskār* (Moon Salutations) is a great way to start your day. Sun Salutations warm and build muscle, while Moon Salutations cool and ground the body. This activity further helps to balance the energies of the body.

- Perform other exercises as desired.

4. Meditate. Lying in *Śavāsana*, or Corpse Pose, is an excellent way to end your morning yoga routine. You can also spend quiet moments sitting and absorbing the smells and sounds around you. This action helps to purify the mind, decluttering it and practicing presence.

5. Eat a sensible breakfast. For optimal benefit, eat according to *Āyurvedic* seasons, times of day, and your personal energetic constitution (*prakṛti*).

How you spend the rest of your day is up to your desires and needs. However, make sure to sustain yourself with good nutrition. A plant-based diet is the cleanest diet. Even if you partake in eating meat, make sure your food sources are raised responsibly. The point to clean living is to keep your footprint small. Do no harm to your food source (*ahiṃṣā*), and your food source will support your health.

The following ideas are also positive changes you can incorporate into your self-care routine:

- Limit the use of technology, especially before bedtime.

- Participate in an evening routine that supports good sleep habits.

- Observe yourself during times of distress or discomfort. Act in a manner that keeps your mind clear, your body pure, and your emotional states calm.

Saṁtoṣa (Contentment)

> *"By contentment, supreme joy is gained."*
> *-The Yoga Sūtra of Patāñjali, 2.42*

Saṁtoṣa is the second *niyama*, designed to help one live in contentment and peace. The underlying concept here is to not simply strive for happiness or satisfaction; the objective is to be content with what happens in life. Be content as you are. Be content with what happens. Of course, if you observe a dysfunctional behavior within yourself, then change that. However, contentment cannot be changed from anything outside of yourself: money, weather, interpersonal relationships, etc. These things cannot change your happiness. If your heart-mind is undisturbed (by following the *yama*s and *niyama*s) and you maintain your body, then contentment will come to you.

Saṁtoṣa occurs when we accept and are content with who we are and what is happening. We can become content when we detach from expectations and certain desired results. *Soham* means "I am That" in Sanskrit. In other words, it is what it is, and I am what I am. Keep this beautiful phrase in your pocket for such an occasion, repeating this mantra to help you in this process.

How to Practice Contentment

- Practice gratitude. Keep a gratitude journal. Share your appreciation with those around you. Say a prayer for all that you are grateful for.

- Be reasonable with your expectations or release them completely. Accept the results for what they are.

- Observe the times when you are dissatisfied with an end result. How can you change the outcome? Either learn to accept it, change your attitude (internal change) or change the circumstance.

- Find blessings in everything, including so-called negative events. When you find the blessing in everything, negative and positive begin to disappear and everything occurs as it is.

- Do not conform to others' mental constructs of what should be. This is especially important while practicing yoga. You do not need to wear certain clothes, own certain accessories, twist your body into painful postures, or meditate for hours while dismissing everything else. Do what works for you and be content.

Tapas (Practice Causing Positive Change)

"By austerity, impurities of body and senses are destroyed and occult powers gained."
-The Yoga Sūtra of Patañjali, 2.43

Tapas is like śauca (with a hint of *samtosā*). However, *tapas*, which means "to burn", is more than simple cleanliness. *Tapas* is to purge, to experience pain, discomfort, and pressure. It is the necessary and uncomfortable changes a person must go through—physically, mentally, and emotionally—to become clean and to find contentment.

When we allow the pain, or put in another way, when we observe our shadow, we can learn to embrace it and slowly detach from any negative judgements. This behavior is austerity in action. Living more simply (doing without), fasting, and experiencing some level of strict scarcity will help to purify the heart-mind and body, but it will also strengthen your ability to accept life as it comes.

How to Practice Causing Positive Change

- Embrace discomfort. Break out of a routine (especially an unhealthy one) for a few days. Observe your physical, mental, and emotional attachment to it.

- Push yourself. Participate in an exercise (or *āsana*!) and work a part of your body harder than you are used to. Speak up about something you've wanted to say. Clean a part of your house you haven't touched in a while. The heat produced from these events will serve as practice in action.

- When you interact with difficult people or observe an undesirable trait within yourself, think of the occurrence as necessary for growth. Heat works to clean and remove impurities.

Svādhyāya (Independent Study)

"By study of spiritual books comes communion with one's chosen deity."
-The Yoga Sūtra of Patāñjali, 2.44

It is okay if you do not partake in religion or choose to study a deity (or maybe you study a variety). Spiritual practice does, however, require serious study. It is through such study that one can participate in self-inquiry and learn important meditative/spiritual techniques and mantras.

This practice in action will lead to many personal insights. It is through these insights that we can observe our imperfections and aspects of ourselves that we want to improve.

Study leads to self-observation. Whether you read poetry, scripture, or self-help books, you will learn about the human condition. It is through this learning that you may adopt rituals for yourself or identify behaviors in which you wish to espouse (or behaviors you wish to avoid). Continuous study and participation in your own spiritual practices can lead you to live in those practices.

How to Practice Independent Study

- Read ancient texts. These include the Bible, Quran, Talmud, Bhagavad Gītā, Tao Te Ching, Vedas, the *Yoga Sūtras*, etc. You may wish to participate in reading works by the saints and practitioners of these religious texts as well.

- If you are not a religious person, find scripture that works for you. Studying does not mean you have to participate in that religion. It means that you are open to its teachings and want to learn for personal growth.

- Adopt a mantra and use it throughout the day. Mantras can help you to connect with the source of your inspiration.

- Through independent study, focus on your own behaviors. Take note of undesirable habits or places in which you wish to improve.

Īśvara-Praṇidhāna (Humility and Faith)

"By total surrender to God, Samādhi is attained."
-The Yoga Sūtra of Patāñjali, 2.45

The meaning of the last *niyama* is to surrender to that which we cannot understand, explain, or find in all our practice. Even people who do not believe in God will find peace in the underlying premise of this *Sūtra*. Our physical body and mental functions are limited to the laws of this world. However, phenomena exist that cannot be explained. When we drop the ego and incessant mind chatter, we recognize that we do not have all the answers. It is through belief and surrender to a higher power that one can attain the ultimate goal of yoga: total absorption and bliss (*Samādhi*, the last limb of *Aṣṭāṅga Yoga*).

This form of surrender helps the human to let go of attachments to earthly desires, live beyond the scope of ego, and helps the heart-mind to see the divine spark in everything. Humility requires acceptance, and faith requires belief. Both of these actions in practice require complete dedication to that with which we owe our existence. In all times, everything can be a teacher and an object of our gratitude for growth. Whether that entity is God or your teachers does not matter. What matters is the surrender and removing yourself as the source of your own greatness.

How to Practice Humility and Faith

- Give credit to your deity (or deities or teachers) for who you have become. You cannot claim your own creation, whether physical, mental, or spiritual. Be proud of your path, but do not let your pride inflate your ego. This action is humility.

- Let go of expectations and trust that everything you need will be provided. See the people in your life as put there for a purpose, even if someone has hurt you. See the blessing in everything, as a divine gift.

- Learn how to see the light of the divine in everyone and everything. It will improve how you treat others, but it will also help you to live in alignment with your own divine nature.

Many paths exist to enlightenment. In *Aṣṭāṇga Yoga*, the practice of one limb (or part of one limb, one *sūtra*) can lead to transformation. It is through the practice of cleanliness that we honor our vessel while realizing its impermanence. It is through the practice of contentment that we maintain internal peace regardless of external circumstances. It is through the practice of causing positive change that we burn away the discomforts and imperfections of ourselves. It is through the practice of independent study that we become more self-aware of our behavior and cultivate a desire to change. It is through the practice of humility and faith that we connect with powers outside of our egos, surrendering to the infinitely possible. Learn, observe, and grow.

3

Pratipakṣa Bhāvana: How to Navigate Conflicting World-views and Build Relationships with Anyone

"When disturbed by negative thoughts, opposite [positive] ones should be thought of. This is pratipakṣa bhāvana."
-The Yoga Sūtra of Patāñjali, 2.33

We live in a world of conflicting viewpoints. And with the aid of technology, these opinions are easily shared (and just as easily instigative). Every person has a unique experience that informs his or her opinions, and this individuality should be celebrated. Unfortunately, information sources aren't concerned about individuality as a way to bless the bounty of this planet—many sources see separation and division as the path toward power, not union.

The intentions of some can easily be the downfall of many. It is in the best interest of certain political leaders and business owners to sway the public to believe in what they are selling. Whether it be legislation, armed conflict, or spending billions of public funds, politicians are increasingly using the media to make people see their "truth." In the same way, business owners use consumer psychology to sell their products and convince the public that their business is essential for quality living. Although many politicians and business owners mean well, some use dishonesty and divisive rhetoric to further bolster their own power. And it is here that we see the effects of *vitarka*.

In Śrī Svāmī Saccidānanda's translation of "The Yoga Sūtras of Patāñjali," *vitarka* translates to "negative thoughts" or "arguments". However, the general Sanskrit translation is "applied attention." Its application refers to debating, discussing, and discursive processes. In Buddhism, the *Vitarka Mudrā* is a hand gesture (thumb and forefinger touching, while the other three fingers point up, palm facing outward near the chest) that denotes debating and discussing teachings. During discourse or the presentation of information, the yoga practitioner must practice *pramāṇa*, which means "correct perception". We must view the information with a clear lens.

Yoga is the practice of clarifying the heart-mind. It is removing the debris and distractions for clear thinking, which leads to clear *Being*. To gain the "correct perception", one must evaluate sources of knowledge thoroughly, using

- Direct perception (*pratyakṣa*)

- Inference (*anumāna*)

- Scriptural testimony (*agamah*)

It is through these reference points that we can prevent misperception, which can lead to suffering by means of violence, theft, and dishonesty. When we dedicate our heart-mind to the Truth, without distraction, we can protect and heal our most treasured personal relationships, but also cultivate relationships with "the other".

How Misinformation Creates Conflict

To practice yoga means to clear the heart-mind (and body) of obstructions (*kleśas*). One of the greatest obstacles to overcome is managing misinformation. The human brain has many jobs, but its largest responsibility is to filter sensory input and then respond accordingly. The sensory organs (skin, nose, eyes, ears, tongue, etc.) receive stimulation by means of touch, temperature, pressure, smell, sight, sound, and taste, and then the associated nerves send messages to the brain about what it is we are experiencing. In an instant, the central nervous system must decide how to use that information to keep the body alive. The nervous system is designed in such a complete way that it can determine whether we need to run away, prepare to fight, or enjoy the ride that is life. But because of our animal instincts, that have been developing for millions of years, we don't immediately see the pleasure in all circumstances.

Since the human mind is designed to survive, we humans have developed what experts call a Negativity Bias. Because surviving seems to be more important than enjoying life, we typically see the world through a lens that actively seeks out negative experiences. We are always on high alert and this influence can cloud our judgment, making us reactive rather than responsive. Often, this important yet primitive way of assessing the environment can negatively impact how humans view the world and its other inhabitants.

With the advancements of the 21st Century, the human mind is less concerned with basic human survival and more with constructing meaning, developing bonds with others, and living according to purpose. Today, we use information and critical thinking skills to determine how we live our lives. Every day, we face massive amounts of information from the Internet, books, radio, podcasts, television, advertisements, and literally any input that finds its way to the sensory organs. And with so much material readily accessible, anyone can share the information, adding their perspective, and creating a new "reality." Many individuals and organizations use this access to share their own vision of reality. Some sincerely want to improve the world, but others have more self-serving motives.

> *"The sources of right knowledge are direct perception,*
> *inference, and scriptural testimony."*
> The Yoga Sūtra of Patāñjali, 1.7

Not all information is created equally. Each source of information has an intention: selling a product or service; selling an idea to further a goal; selling a political platform for election; etc. Some intentions are noble and meant to improve life, using the principles of Love, Beauty, and Truth. However, some intentions are self-serving, meant to further the source's personal power and wealth. Because the information we receive may not be rooted in truth (*satya*), may intend to cause harm (*ahiṃsā*), or may deplete precious resources (*asteya*), the mind and heart can become cloudy and maligned intentions can leave a negative impression. For this reason, the heart-mind must be a filter for all incoming information.

Pratyakṣa (Direct Perception)

Often, we do not have the luxury of being a first-hand witness to an event. We must listen to or read about other people's perspectives and take their words at face-value. This faith in others' perspectives can be dangerous. Even the most trustworthy person will retell an event through his or her lens. This lens comes with filters from culture, language, and experiences that differ from yours and from the majority of the world. Imagine for a moment, growing up in a province of China or being a native of Switzerland. How different would your life be from what it is now? Even in the United States, there is a vast difference between people from urban and rural regions, Northern and Southern regions, and East and West Coastal regions. Even neighbors can have vastly different political, religious, or cultural beliefs and practices.

Every person views the world through an individual lens. Every event we've witnessed, word we've heard, smell we've smelled—everything—has had an effect on us. In yoga, these impressions are called *saṁskāras*, and it is the intention of the yogi to eliminate the hold these impressions have on the heart-mind. One way to do this is to understand that every source of information comes from someone else's *saṁskāras*; therefore, it is essential to try and use direct perception as much as possible to filter sensory input:

- Pay more attention to primary sources, especially in the news media. Pay less attention to commentaries on those events.

- Engage in practice. Don't just read about something or listen to others' first-hand accounts. Try the activity.

- Pause for reflection. Take a moment to process what has happened. In yoga *āsana* (practicing physical postures), the last pose is usually *Śavāsana* (Corpse Pose). The intention is to let the mind and body absorb and process what just occurred. In the same way, pause to think about what you just saw, heard, or felt. Try to be objective and empathetic in your witnessing.

Anumāna (Inference)

To infer means to make a logical conclusion based on evidence. In Śrī Svāmī Saccidānanda's translation of this *Sūtra*, he describes a situation where a person can infer there is a fire if he or she sees or smells smoke. That is logical. But the information we receive in the world is a continuous barrage of statements, sounds, and symbols, and it is often difficult to take the time to make inferences. It is easier to just take someone's message as truth. This blind acceptance, however, will lead to damage, as it clouds the mind and makes it difficult to assess the reality of such messages.

Making inferences requires a person to deduce or induce logical confirmations. Deduction moves from theory to hypothesis, and then from observation to confirmation. Using deduction to come to a conclusion is the act of taking general information and coming up with a specific answer. Adversely, induction moves from an observation (say direct perception) to a pattern, and then creating a hypothesis and finally a theory based on that pattern. Using induction to come to a conclusion is the act of taking specific information and coming up with a general answer. In yoga, we can participate in practices, experiment and observe, and see what happens, leading to a general conclusion (induction). We can also see that the general consensus that practicing yoga leads to health and wellness is true by seeing the results in our own mind-bodies and concluding that yoga is the cause (deduction).

Here are some questions to ask yourself when making inferences:

- What do I know about this subject?

- Do I need to learn more?

- What do I know about the source of information?

- Is there a more reliable source?

- Where can I glean reliable information?

To simplify, always ask yourself the who, what, where, when, and especially why of a scenario. Try and look at the situation from someone else's point-of-view. And most importantly, does the story *feel* right? Inference requires the logic of the mind, but the heart, when clear, can also assess a situation based on its moral integrity.

Agamah (Scriptural Testimony)

Scripture, according to Śrī Svāmī Saccidānanda's translation, refers to holy literature brought forth from "sages, saints, and prophets" (p. 12). These words contain universal truths that stand the test of time. No matter where we live or in what time period we dwell, the Golden Rule applies to all creatures, the path to peace consists of parallel practices, and we all derive from the same source. Even if you choose to live separately from one another and build up walls, you cannot deny that we are all from the same material, and when we die, our bodies will break down but will never disappear. It may seem like scriptural texts divide us, but they do the opposite: These ancient words keep us connected and provide wisdom to meet our basic human needs.

We already know that the *Yoga Sūtras* contain guideposts for living in a way that brings contentment. These teachings come from ancient scripture, and this guidance matches the teachings of other traditions:

- Do not steal

- Do no harm

- Do not lie

- Love and treat others as you would want to be treated

- Serve the poor and destitute

- Live presently

- Take responsibility for your actions

We can see these teachings in the Christian Bible, the Hindu Vedas and Upanishads, the Buddhist Tipitaka, the Jewish Talmud and Tanakh, the Muslim Quran, the Shinto Kojiki, and much more. We also see these teachings in "The Yoga Sūtras of Patanjali," which is not a religious text, and we see similar teachings expounded upon by trusted scholars and other sources. Even Atheism, Humanism, and other secular wisdom prescribes certain "truths" to bring us order amidst chaos.

What is *Pramāṇa* and How can it Heal Divides?

"Misconception occurs when knowledge of something is not based upon its true form."
-The Yoga Sūtra of Patāñjali, 1.8

In Sanskrit, *pramāṇa* translates to "means of knowledge". You can think of it as a means of proof. When faced with information, which we intake daily, it is essential to verify its validity. Does it match your direct perceptions of the events? Does it make sense, and can you make logical inferences between what is known and the information? Does it come from a trusted source, based on certain universal truths that are at the foundation of our existence? If the information doesn't match up with reality, then we must act by either denouncing or remaining cautious of the source.

"An image that arises on hearing mere words without any reality [at its basis] is verbal delusion."
-The Yoga Sūtra of Patāñjali, 1.9

Subscribing to delusion is to live in a false world with false perceptions. Believing falsehoods creates an impure lens. Viewing the world and others from this perspective can cause conflict by means of divorce, lost friends, hurt family members, estranged children, and feuding neighbors. If we take it to another level, it can cause strife among nations, which leads to extreme poverty, inhumane treatment and genocide, and endless war.

Loving-Kindness Meditation

When we use diligence, intelligence, and a clear heart-mind to navigate sensory input, we do ourselves and the world a favor by maintaining peace and calm. However, damage may already exist within ourselves, our loved ones, and even our enemies. Although enemies is a strong word, we create them by seeing anyone as "the other". We can heal these divides by practicing the *Yoga Sūtras* described above and by participating in the following Loving-Kindness Meditation, which can be found in "One Simple Thing: A New Look at the Science of Yoga and How it Can Transform Your Life," by Eddie Stern.

Note: *These can be done in one 10-15 minute meditative session, or you can work on each aspect for 1-2 days, completing a week-long cycle (i.e. days 1 and 2, focus on you;*

days 3 and 4, focus on your loved ones; days 5 and 6, focus on strangers; and day 7, focus on a difficult relationship).

1. **Begin by directing loving and forgiving wishes toward yourself.** Repeat each phrase four times, then repeat the process three times:

    May I be safe. May I be happy. May I be healthy. May I be peaceful.

    To whom I have hurt knowingly or unknowingly, I ask forgiveness.

    To those who have hurt me knowingly or unknowingly, I forgive.

    I forgive myself for hurting myself knowingly or unknowingly.

2. **Send forgiving and loving thoughts to those people with whom you feel close.** Imagine a close friend, family member, or someone whom you admire. Visualize this person sending you the above affirmations in a warm and gentle manner. Extend this same action toward this individual, sending them love and support through this meditation.

60

3. **Once you are used to the Loving-Kindness mantras, extol these feelings and wishes to people you don't know:** The postal worker, police officer, a neighbor you've never met, or even someone from another country. You can use these words or create your own mantras based on what feels right.

4. **Lastly, extend these wishes to the "difficult person" or "the other".** It may help to visualize the other person as a vulnerable infant so that they seem less harsh. Remember that like you, they too have suffered, and in turn, you may be just as difficult a person to them as they are to you. If it is too difficult to be warming and compassionate, try to remain neutral. Use universal truths and wisdom to support healing.

As Eddie Stern writes, "When we close our heart, we suffer, and we are the ones who get caught in the snare of sorrow. Loving-kindness works on the relationship without the other person knowing. So we work on our own, and it changes the dynamic of the relationship and leaves room for openness. We don't do it to change the other person; we do it to transform our heart and to release the pain we are carrying. Forgiveness is a good way to release the knot" (p. 269).

4

Śānti: How to Maintain Personal Peace and Power in Relationships

"By cultivating attitudes of friendliness toward the happy, compassion for the unhappy, delight in the virtuous and disregard toward the wicked, the mind-stuff retains its undisturbed calmness."
-The Yoga Sūtra of Patāñjali, 1.33

Relationships can be complicated. We have many different types of relationships: Some are personal and by choice, while others are circumstantial and obligatory. But the truth is that no matter what the circumstance, we all have a choice on how to act and react in regard to the people with whom we experience life.

Relationships among people are important. They provide each of us with a support system, and they can bring joy and happiness to our lives. However, some relationships hurt and diminish the quality of life. While relationships matter, they must not interfere with your personal peace and power.

According to Patañjali's *Sūtra* 1.33, there are four types of people, which will be represented by four locks:

- Happy

- Unhappy

- Virtuous

- Wicked

This is not to say that a happy person cannot also be virtuous, or that wickedness cannot lead to unhappiness. However, these distinctions matter when we think about how to approach different types of people (or different behaviors within one person). Which *key* should we use for which lock?

- Friendliness for the Happy

- Compassion for the Unhappy

- Delight for the Virtuous

- Disregard for the Wicked

We do not use these keys for the benefit of others. Of course, if we practice yoga, we emanate Love. We are Love. And so, when we practice Love, we affect other people. But the point of Patāñjali's words are to promote inner peace—Self Love—to avoid suffering for yourself. Yoga is a process of personal work, which happens to also affect the collective. By practicing this *Sūtra*, you are keeping a serene mind, which is a part of the path of yoga.

Therefore, the interpersonal goal is not to simply maintain a one-size-fits-all approach. The interpersonal goal is to use the tools provided to you through yogic practice—the keys—so that when you meet a lock, it will not disturb your inner peace.

What is Inner Peace and Personal Power?

The intention of yoga practice is to create a unified heart-mind, but the path to reaching union (literal meaning of yoga) is multiform. *Sādhana* is Sanskrit for "spiritual practice." In yoga, *sādhana* is the means to create inner and outer union. It is the multi-faceted and personal approach one takes to live a yogic lifestyle. You must change your inner and outer world to become congruent with a divine consciousness.

A part of this work consists of cultivating conscientious living. According to Patāñjali, there are four aspects of consciousness:

- *Citta* = mind stuff

- *Ahaṃkāra* = ego feeling

- *Buddhi* = discriminative faculty

- *Manas* = the desiring faculty of the mind stuff

Citta is the subjective judgment we place on an experience. The subjective reactions to stimuli can create extreme responses, positive or negative. *Citta* refers to the feelings we associate with experiences, and it is referred to as the mind stuff, or lower mind, because these feelings affect our ego consciousness. To put it plainly, Śrī Svāmī Saccidānanda explains that "*citta* is the sum total of the mind" and is made up of the different levels: *ahaṃkāra* ("basic mind"), *buddhi* ("intellect"), and *manas* (the perceiving mind that "gets attracted to outside things through the senses") (p. 4).

Patāñjali described yoga to neutralize the feelings of the lower mind. Yoga works to still the mind, to elevate the consciousness to one of control, which also includes our reactions to others. *Citta* resides in the heart. When we live

65

by the tenets of yoga, we can learn to calm the temperament of the heart (in this case, our reactions to other people) and observe from a place of "undisturbed calmness" (*Sūtra* 1.33). It is through this inner peace that we gain our composure and power.

The Four Locks: How Other People Choose to Live

Relationships take two people to work. However, the dynamics among our various associations will differ as widely as the people who inhabit the planet. Each person has a different life experience, with a unique set of values, personality traits, and ways of viewing the world. Nevertheless, each person typically exists in one of the four common characteristics mentioned earlier.

It is worth noting here, however, that although each person generally exists within one of these four categories, this *Sūtra* can also help to handle changing relationship issues in the moment. For example: A generally happy person may experience a period of unhappiness, or that toddler who always shares her toys may experience bouts of temporary wickedness.

When we approach these people, whether just meeting them or engaging with a lifelong partner, it is important to determine which lock they are, because the inner work you do for yourself will always provide you with the key.

Happy People

According to Patañjali, the first lock is happy people (*sukha*). In Sanskrit, *sukha* means "happiness". Happy people emanate joy. They are recognizable by their smiles and their pleasant demeanor. They may or may not have a reason to be happy, but they are. Even in moments of sadness, grief, or anger, they seem to exude a sense of overall contentment in life. Happy people come from a place of acceptance and gratitude.

Unhappy People

The second lock is unhappy people (*duḥkha*). In Sanskrit, *duḥkha* translates to "suffering". Unhappy people always have something to complain about. They seem to attract unpleasant circumstances, as they typically believe life is full of hardship. Even in a moment of pleasure, they are sure to focus on an aspect they deem negative. Instead of gratitude for their circumstances, unhappy people feel slighted. Overall, unhappy people come from a place of criticism and blame.

Virtuous People

The third lock is the virtuous (*puṇya*). In Sanskrit, *puṇya* translates directly to "virtuous". These people are generous and philanthropic by nature. They are typically pillars of the community and use their lives to serve others. They may be happy in their virtue, but their overall effect on others is through their excellent behavior and service.

Wicked People

The fourth lock is the wicked (*apuṇya*). In Sanskrit, *apuṇya* means non-virtuous. The translation from Śrī Svāmī Saccidānanda refers to the unvirtuous as wicked. These may be people who live an overall amoral life, or they may actively participate in destructive behavior. The wicked among us have inflated egos and typically act in a way to serve only themselves. People can also act this way temporarily, especially during moments of desperation or as a means of obtaining power.

The Four Keys: How You Choose to Live

A yogic lifestyle will provide you with the tools to maintain a calm heart-mind. Think about the center, your core, as being a pond. Stimuli will cause a response, ripples.

Practicing yoga will help to decrease the volatility of these ripples, if not eliminate them altogether. Through consistent practice, you can become disciplined in a way to keep an undisturbed heart-mind, regardless of the actions of others.

Sūtra 2.12 explains how obstacles (*kleśas*) create the tendencies (*saṁskāras*) that affect our actions and their outcomes (*karma*). Negative reactions and emotions are afflictions of the heart-mind and lead to undesirable consequences. The five *kleśas* are as follows:

- *Avidyā* = lack of awareness

- *Asmitā* = egotism, feeling more or less than others

- *Rāga* = desire for prior pleasures

- *Dveṣa* = aversion to prior pain

- *Abbiniveśa* = fear of death, attachment to life

Nicolai Bachman explains, in his book "The Path of the Yoga Sūtras: A Practical Guide to the Core of Yoga", the necessity of weakening these obstacles to promote inner peace. It is the *kleśas* that cause us to suffer, to lack inner peace. We can gain power over them by diminishing their potency (by controlling our emotional reactions). Through practicing positive change (*tapas*), self-observation (*svādhyāya*), and humility with faith (*Īśvara-Praṇidhāna*), we can provide the discipline required for an undisturbed heart-mind.

Friendliness

When you come across someone who is happy, meet them with friendliness. *Maitrī* is the Sanskrit word for "friendliness", which is the key to *sukha*. But why would you need a key when in the presence of someone who is happy? Remember, yoga is about personal peace. This *Sūtra* relates to our reactions to others. When we see someone who is happy, we must be friendly toward that person to maintain an undisturbed heart-mind. It is possible to be jealous or annoyed by people who are happy. Negative emotions can arise when we observe another's abundance. In this moment, act friendly toward the happy, and you will preserve inner peace.

Compassion

It is easy to judge people who are unhappy. It is common to express frustration with someone's actions, blaming them for their own discontent. Their unhappiness is the result of their actions (*karma*), so why should you help them? Or maybe it is within your nature to try and fix the situation, to dole out advice, even when your advice is not sought.

In these instances, use compassion (*karunā*) as your key. Meet someone who is unhappy with understanding, love, and mercy. Don't blame them. Don't belittle them. Don't chastise them or try and change their situation. Help them the way you can, either with your time, talents, or physical necessities. Sit with the unhappy and listen to their grieving hearts. Provide them with the unconditional love that comes from your being. By acting in this way, you are taking responsibility for your actions. Compassion is also the path to self-awareness and can be a mirror to our own behavior.

Delight

As with happy people, it is possible to experience jealousy or disdain when in the presence of the virtuous. Sometimes, the virtuous are also people with whom you disagree. If someone identifies with a different religion, political belief system, or other core value, yet they perform righteous acts, delight in their virtue.

Delight (*muditā*) is the key to *punya*. And not only should you find joy in their generosity—mind, body, and spirit—but you should also work to act in a similar manner. Use your moral compass to do good. In what ways can you act virtuously? If you live according to the *Yoga Sūtras* and follow the eight-limbed path, then you will find it natural to share light with those around you.

Disregard

This key may be the most difficult to use, but it can be the most liberating. The wicked act in ways that hurt others. They may generally espouse amoral or even abusive behavior, or they act in a manner that is temporarily troublesome. Regardless, the key to *apuṇya* is disregard (*upekṣā*).

Again, you may attempt to treat an unvirtuous person in the same way you would an unhappy person by trying to tell them how they should live. While acting this way with an unhappy person can disturb your peace, because your advice may fall upon deaf ears, acting this way with a wicked person can destroy your life.

Here is an anecdote that Śrī Svāmī Saccidānanda shares in his translation of *Sūtra* 1.33, which illuminates the ways of the wicked:

> A monkey sits upon a branch, out in the rain. Across from him is a beautiful sparrow nest. Sparrows' nests are known for their

elaborate inner workings: They build rooms
that provide shelter for all who inhabit it.
Well, on this day, the sparrow peaked out
from her nest and saw the monkey. She tried
to understand why the monkey could not
do what she had done. She asked the
monkey why he would allow himself to get
wet, being that he was a distant cousin to
humans and capable of much more.
Monkeys have hands for creating such a
dwelling, while sparrows merely have beaks.
She pointed out her own work, her own
inner peace.

The monkey reacted as the wicked react. He
tore up her nest, destroying every inch of it.
He resented her for her words and berated
her with insults.

There is nothing the sparrow could have done in this
situation, except disregard the monkey from the beginning.
It is the same way with many people we encounter. They
may seem unhappy, or pretend to be happy or even
virtuous, but when someone tries to help them or give them
advice, they lash out. They are the wicked, because they
destroy what is around them. They will destroy your inner
peace and dismantle your personal power. Stay away from

them. If you cannot avoid them, disregard their unscrupulous behavior and hurtful words.

How to Use these Keys to Maintain Peace and Power

In this life, you will meet many different people. You will experience these encounters briefly, or they will develop into lasting relationships. Regardless, your commitment and responsibility is to your heart-mind. The yogic lifestyle will assist you in understanding how your actions create consequences (your *karma*, the ripples in your pond). In dealing with people, your goal is to maintain your peace and composure. You cannot get lost or allow your lower-mind to become disturbed.

Be friendly toward the happy and compassionate toward the unhappy. Take delight in the virtuous and emulate their example. Disregard the wicked and retain your inner calm in the face of their actions.

The practice of yoga will prepare you to use these keys. It will help you to become more aware and to recognize the four locks: *sukha*, *duḥkha*, *puṇya*, and *apuṇya*. The yogic lifestyle will also help you to react to these circumstances in a way that will not disturb your wellbeing and peace.

Through *maitrī*, *karunā*, *muditā*, and *upekṣā*, your heart-mind will remain calm, and your peace will remain undisturbed.

5

Samādhi: How the Inner Journey toward Self will Bring You Closer to the Divine Consciousness

"By total surrender to God, Samādhi is attained."
-The Yoga Sūtra of Patāñjali, 2.45

Some say that relationship is the meaning of life. We are in relationship with every ecosystem on the planet, at the macro and micro levels. From the stars and planets to Earth and her inhabitants, we are connected to all. It is through the journey of yoga that we can build and strengthen these relationships, eventually experiencing a great sense of joy through unity.

To practice yoga is to travel inward from the world outside to the ultimate internal wisdom that all exists as a unified consciousness. As humans, we relate to this transcendence in four stages, which can correlate to the connections we share through relationship:

- Reason and our relationship with gross objects in the outside world

- Reflection and our relationship with ideas and experiences closer to our heart-mind

- Rejoicing and our relationship with ourselves

- Pure "I-am-ness" and our relationship with supreme consciousness or God

It is in this final stage that we can experience the ultimate union, where the individual becomes completely absorbed and connected to the Source of all. Described in the *Yoga Sūtras*, bliss, nirvana, or supreme joy is experienced through actualizing the "supreme *Puruṣa*", or "supreme Self" (p. 37). This special Self is the Divine, God, Spirit, Universal or Collective Consciousness, Awareness, Source, or any other term used for the entity that is in us all that experiences no attachment or affliction. Patāñjali calls this supreme soul *Īśvara*, which in Sanskrit translates to "supreme God".

The supreme soul that Patāñjali describes is not "out there"; "Heaven" is not a place we go after death. The individual soul (each person) is not separate from the supreme soul. We are all divine consciousness manifested as unique beings. The journey of yoga is inward. With each action, the practitioner works to prepare and purify the body and mind. By practicing *Yama, Niyama, Āsana, Prānāyāma, Pratyāhāra, Dhāraṇā, and Dhyāna,* one may experience that journey, eventually reaching *Samādhi.*

What is *Samādhi* and How Can it Lead to Relationship with the Divine?

Samādhi is the eighth and final limb of *Aṣṭāṅga Yoga.* It is not the objective or the goal; the purpose of yoga is in the journey. However, it is in *Samādhi* that the practitioner can experience liberation from all attachment and union with all.

As described many times in this book, yoga means "union"; therefore, its practice leads unity on many levels. First, the individual aligns with divine Truth, Beauty, and Love through the *yama-s* and *niyama.* Second, the body and breath align with one another through *āsana* and *prānāyāma* to create union with the body and mind. This action further creates unity through *pratyahara,* as the mind's increased and steady focus shuts off external sensory input. This direct focus leads the practitioner deeper into *dhāraṇā* and *dhyāna,* both meditative states that allow the mind to detach from the world outside and into a state of unity consciousness. It is in a state of complete attention, "total dedication" (p. 37), that one can experience *Samādhi*.

In Sanskrit, *Samādhi* means "to collect" or "direct together." The process is achieved through complete absorption and transcendence. The individual is no longer the individual, as union is achieved through deep meditation and focus. The result is a deep sense of joy, as the meditator, the meditated upon, and even the process of meditation all become one reality. This union feels like bliss, because it is actualizing God—one's true essence.

Although this is the progression of *Aṣṭāṅga Yoga*, there is no one way to achieve *Samādhi*. Initially, it is an eventual gradation, because you have to train the mind to enter the subtle body and then remove all objects completely (including the Self). However, some individuals can experience *Samādhi* instantly with focus. Some of us will even experience glimpses of *Samādhi* when we lose ourselves in a task or moment. Think about a time when you've concentrated so intently on a task that you become one with it. This can happen while cleaning, creating art, dancing, or other processes. All time seems to slip away; sounds, smells, external sights, and other sensory perception disappear as the mind becomes one with the moment.

And, of course, it occurs in meditation. This process is broken down further into two types of *Samādhi: samprajñāta (*distinguished) and *asamprajñāta* (undistinguished). *Asamprajñāta* occurs after experiencing the various stages of *samprajñāta*:

- *Savitarka Samādhi* (concentration on gross objects or *prakṛiti*)

- *Savicāra Samādhi* (concentration on subtle elements (*tanmātras*) or mind-stuff (*citta*)

- *Sa-ānanda Samādhi* (concentration of *sattvic* mind devoid of any object other than joy)

- *Sa-asmita Samādhi* ("I" feeling alone)

In the various stages of *samprajñāta Samādhi*, the impressions (*samskāras*) of mental modifications still exist. The mind is still aware of something, even if it is only of the absolute awareness of being one with all. Beyond this is *asamprajñāta Samādhi*, in which no impressions or "buried seeds" (p. 33) exist. Here there is only supreme consciousness. The stages of *samprajñāta* prepare the practitioner by understanding *Prakṛiti* (matter, energy, Nature), being able to put all of it aside in order to live in a liberated state, free from attachment. There is nothing

80

obstructing the mind: "You understand yourself to be the pure Self, or the *Puruṣa,* which seemed to have been entangled in *Prakṛiti* and is now finally free" (p. 34).

However, to achieve this liberation, one must truly comprehend that which must be transcended. It is during the distinguished layers of *Samādhi* (*saṁprajñāta*) that the mind experiences four progressions to the essential "I am ness". Its layers are more concrete and progress, because as Śrī Svāmī Saccidānanda explains, "...you can't immediately contemplate the very subtle. First you have to train the mind to focus on something concrete" (p. 30). This first level of absolute focus is *savitarka Samādhi.*

Savitarka Samādhi

The first level of *Samādhi* is *savitarka,* which refers to thoughtfulness or contemplation. To understand the subtle energies, one must first understand the gross elements, or *prakṛiti.* This term refers to energy, the basic organic material from which all matter is created. When it is capitalized, as Patāñjali often does, it refers to the world. In the beginning was unmanifested, unorganized matter.

Regardless of one's beliefs about creation, it is impossible to disregard the realities of matter: It cannot be destroyed, and it cannot be created. It is anything that is composed of atomic material and has mass; therefore, every gross object that we can sense (see, smell, touch, taste, hear) is composed of this energy.

After choosing to focus upon a concrete object (*dhāraṇā*) and continually focusing upon it (*dhyāna*) one will eventually begin to understand it at its most elemental level. Here you can study, contemplate, and understand an object: a flame, a rock, a pattern, etc. In this most fundamental step toward training the mind, the practitioner begins to understand every aspect of the concrete object.

Tanmātras Samādhi

Tanmātras is a reflective state. This next progression refers to the subtle essence of matter, the abstract. Here the practitioner contemplates an intangible quality or concept, like the color green or the principles of truth. This type of concentration and understanding is difficult to achieve if one does not have the mental expansion built through *savitarka Samādhi*.

It is the same with *āsana* or *prāṇāyāma*: It is impossible to perform certain physical poses if the body is not in shape, or for the lungs to perform certain breathwork if they do not have the capacity to retain the breath for longer periods. Once one builds the mental capacity to understand many concrete objects, then one can begin to contemplate and truly understand the qualities of abstract concepts. The practitioner is Green. The practitioner is Truth. All the qualities inherent in these concepts are inherent in all consciousness.

Savicāra Samādhi

Savicāra is an even simpler form of meditation, although it is more difficult to achieve and explain. Here, the practitioner does not meditate upon an object or concept; the practitioner contemplates the mind. It is important for the mind to evolve and involve containing the capacity for this level of *Samādhi*. Once one is in this state, the mind is at peace. That is why this is the state of rejoicing. The mind is tranquil and capable of rejoicing in its own being. Only joy and tranquility exist in this stage of *Samādhi*, there is "no reasoning or reflection" (p. 31).

Sa-asmita Samādhi

Sa-asmita is to contemplate pure "I-am-ness". In this state, the practitioner is not even aware of the mind, itself, just the "I". It is a presence without anything else present. You are. That is all.

Relationship and Unity Consciousness

As the practitioner travels further inward, the process
becomes less descriptive, because there is less "mind-stuff"
or *citta* to process. Patañjali explains the gradual growing
capacity of the heart-mind to reach the pure "I-am-ness"
that is *sa-asmita Samādhi* and the supreme soul
(God/Īśvara). The process leads one to God, because it is in
this process that one can see the divine in all beings. Once a
person can identify and appreciate the divine in all, he or she
can immediately achieve (and even live in) a state of
Samādhi. Although this direct *Samādhi* is unusual, it is the
goal of yoga: to live in a state of union, recognizing the
divine manifest in everything.

Total Surrender to God (*Īśvara Praṇidhānā*)

Before continuing down this journey, let me be clear: The
faith and return to Source described in the *Yoga Sūtras* is
personal. Whether an individual practices Buddhism,
Hinduism, Christianity, Judaism, or some other spiritual
path, or if an individual is agnostic or undecided, the point
of yoga is not to find the distinction among the various
beliefs. Union does not separate; it tears down boundaries
and unites. It is impossible to reach this level of absolute
liberation without meeting the divine light that resides in all

beings. Afterall, *namaste* translates to "I bow to the divine light in you." If you are not ready to agree to a universal God or any higher power altogether, that is okay. But in practicing yoga, with discipline and dedication, it is impossible not to arrive at this union. It is what you will find on the journey.

Īśvara praṇidhānā is complete dedication to God, and since God is in everything, the practitioner dedicates their life to all. In this way, any communication can become prayer, any task a sacred ritual, and any space an altar. Śrī Svāmī Saccidānanda provides several examples to illuminate the importance of service to everything, in every moment, even inanimate objects and mundane chores. Whatever we handle in a crude or rough manner, will screech, crack, or respond with dissonance. Whatever we choose to move, clean, or maintain in a gentle manner, will respond with ease and harmony. We can feel tremendous joy, even in the maintenance of inanimate objects. Imagine how glorious it would feel to provide this love and care to living creatures! This is dedication to God.

When we live in this dedication, it brings us a great sense of peace, because complete dedication means that we have let go of all attachments. *Samādhi* is a state in which we live in total dedication to the supreme soul. We can do this through meditation, expansion of the mind, and removal of attachment (judgements, fears, desires, etc.). We can also dedicate our lives through service.

Faith in Action (*Dharma*)

Samādhi can be attained through meditation, yes, but it is given life through serving others. According to Seane Corn's "Revolution of the Soul," *Samādhi* is "seeing equally". It is accepting what is, living in the present, and removing all attachment to desires of the mind—what should have been, what should be, how it should be, etc. In order to Be in this state of liberation, it is essential to identify one's purpose and freely give this gift. Come as you are.

The soul's work is called *dharma*. This is the rawest and most essential aspect of any manifestation of life. *Dharma* is seeing your calling and committing to using that call to benefit others. The purpose of answering the call is to evolve the collective consciousness. This is serious dedication to God.

There is a story about Gautam Buddha's death and approach to the gates of Heaven. He sees all the enlightened beings on the other side, but he chooses not to enter: He is waiting for the remainder of humanity to become liberated. He will be the last to enter the Kingdom. In the same way, the teachings of Jesus highlight love, service, and non-attachment to worldly possessions. Above all, treat others as yourself. The *Bhagavad Gītā* says, "By total dedication, unending peace" (as quoted in *Yoga Sūtra* 2.45).

Śrī Svāmī Saccidānanda explains that it doesn't matter what religion, philosophy, or path one takes, all means of dedication to God reach the same outcome. The teachings of those who dedicate their lives to God share one common mission: Shine your light onto all. Give of yourself. See this light, the light of God in all. Be the change this world desperately needs. Keep in the work and wait at the gates while all the world finds its liberation.

And one does not need to be a strict yoga practitioner to find *Samādhi*. Purifying one's heart-mind through any practice: Dedicating your life to the virtues through the *yamas* and *niyamas*; the discipline of *āsana* and *prāṇāyāma*; or the mindful and gentle focus of *pratyāhāra, dhāraṇā,* and *dhyāna* will provide peace to the individual soul. And this soul will act in such a way, that it will change the world.

II

The Yogic Lifestyle:
A Foundation
for Health

1

Āsana: The Health Benefits of a Physical Practice (On and Off the Mat)

"Āsana is a steady, comfortable posture."
-The Yoga Sūtra of Patāñjali, 2.46

Yoga is an ancient way of living, established with the intention of achieving union—the union of the physical, mental, and spiritual bodies in each of us, as well as union with divine consciousness. Ultimately, union can be achieved through *Samādhi*, which is a complete absorption with no distractions, boundaries, or conflicts. The yoga practitioner refines the many layers of the body to reach *Samādhi* but to also improve everyday life.

Āsana, which refers to the physical practice of yoga, is a pathway toward refining the body and mind. Immediate benefits of participating in *āsana* include:

- Regulating stress

- Releasing toxins stored in the body

- Allowing life force energy (*prāṇa*) to flow

The long-term effects of a consistent yoga practice are even more rewarding:

- Increasing stamina

- Creating supple joints and muscles

- Decreasing back and body pain

- Elongating the spine (and reversing the effects of gravity)

- Establishing a stronger core

- Improving organ function to include major body systems and the vagus nerve

While the body benefits from *āsanas*, practicing yoga also benefits mental and spiritual health through increasing awareness, attention, and personal growth. Its practice aids in keeping the subtle body (the *cakras*) clear for optimizing energy and healing. And the best part is that these benefits continue off the mat by improving daily life through work productivity, cultivating interpersonal relationships, and maintaining life balance. These benefits lead to contentment, personal peace, and joy.

What is *Āsana* and How Does it Benefit Health?

Engaging in *āsana* is to participate in the eight-limbed process of *Aṣṭāṅga Yoga*. *Āsana* is the third limb, necessary to the entire process. What follows is *Prāṇāyāma* (breath control), *Pratyāhāra* (sensory withdrawal), *Dhāraṇā* (concentration), *Dhyāna* (meditation), and *Samādhi* (absorption). These five limbs are the meditative qualities of achieving union though yoga practice. *Āsana* refines the body so that the practitioner can meditate without worrying about the burdens of the body.

In Patāñjali's *Yoga Sūtras*, *āsana* refers to the posture that we use during seated meditation. In Sanskrit, *āsana* translates to "seat". However, as the term has evolved, *āsana* also refers to physical yoga practice and its postures. The objective of practicing the various postures is to be able to "sit" comfortably for longer periods of time. Initially, practitioners of meditation found that they could not sit for long periods of time without discomfort. Their constant shifting and aches interfered with their meditation. The origins of *Hatha Yoga* developed *āsana* over time as a way to combat this interference. First, early practitioners focused on their diet. Second, they worked on eliminating the various toxins in the body through bending, twisting, and squeezing the body and its organs.

How Diet Affects *Āsana*

The body is a chemical factory. It produces its own chemicals, such as hormones, neurotransmitters, and other substances that allow the body to function. Imbalances (deficiencies and excess levels) of any substance can cause harm to the body. These problems can manifest into pain, stiffness, and organ disease (dis-ease). Sometimes the body has natural deficiencies or surpluses, but sometimes poor diet and exercise can create imbalances. By paying attention to nutrient intake and activity level, a person can combat the effects of toxins in the body.

Āyurveda is the sister science of yoga, and it means "knowledge of life". This knowledge includes using food as medicine to heal the body. The practitioner must learn what to eat and when to eat. To live an *Āyurvedic* lifestyle is to embrace your natural energy composition and then cure what is imbalanced. The underlying principle is that opposites cure, and this healing is achieved through eating seasonally, eating meals that balance your specific constitution, and eating consistent meals during different times of the day.

Although this is a simplified explanation of *Āyurveda*, it is not difficult to use food in a way that supports *āsana* and the other limbs of *Aṣṭāṅga Yoga*. The key is to eat the right foods, in the right quantities, and at the right times:

- Use awareness of food qualities by enjoying a *sattvic* diet. This diet consists of eating foods that enhance mental clarity and physical health through limiting toxins. *Sattvic* food comes from sources that are seasonally harvested, produced in ethical ways, and are mostly organic and plant based. However, consuming meat and dairy is okay, if you choose, as long as the products come from protected animals.

- A core *sattvic* diet should consist of mild foods that are rich in nutrients, such as legumes, whole grains, nuts and seeds, herbal teas, and plants (fruits and vegetables). A *sattvic* diet consists of eating these foods in moderation.

- Avoid or limit foods that are *rajasic* or *tamasic*. *Rajasic* foods include hot spices and stimulants, such as caffeine. These are okay in moderation and when ingested at the right time. *Tamasic* foods come from unsustainable or non-ethical food sources. Meat sourced from violent environments (always practice *ahiṁsā*), alcohol, and processed food are examples of *tamasic* food sources.

- Do not overeat (even *sattvic* foods) and eat during the right times of the day (early morning, noon, and no later than 6 in the evening).

When yoga practitioners are mindful about their diets and use the principles above, they can enjoy a body that can participate more efficiently in *āsana*. Toxins can manifest through gastrointestinal issues, such as bloating, gas, or acid reflux, as well as sluggishness and headaches. Pay attention to foods that cause these problems and try to avoid them. In the same way, eat foods that make you feel great.

How Postures Affect *Āsana*

Although yoga has become popularized as physical exercise with many health benefits, its application has been misunderstood. A traditional yoga practice is intended to move the body in specific ways that help the body eliminate toxins so that the practitioner can sit more comfortably in meditation. With the right postures (again, can be referred to as *āsana*), one can reap the benefits of yoga in a way that

94

improves mental, emotional/spiritual, and physical health. And of course, this step leads the practitioner down the path of the eight limbs.

The Breath

- Each movement must coordinate with the breath. Slow, deliberate movements will help you achieve this task. Typically, the body inhales on upward and expansive movements, while the body exhales during downward and constrictive movements.

- The consciousness of breath should be directed toward the part of the body being manipulated (through twisting, bending, etc.). This further helps the mind concentrate so the body and mind can better achieve union.

The Postures

Different postures exist to have different effects on the body. Expansive and elongated poses should be countered by constrictive poses, and vice versa. Regardless of the amount of time on the mat or the ability of the practitioner, each yoga practice should include poses that move the spine in six ways: forward, backward, laterally (side to side), and twisting each way.

- **Standing Poses:** These poses enhance strength, balance, flexibility, and stamina. The joints and muscles benefit. Common standing *āsana* includes *Tāḍāsana* (Mountain Pose), *Vṛkṣāsana* (Tree Pose), and *Vīrabhadrāsana* I, II, III (Warrior Poses 1, 2, 3). Standing poses are typically the easiest for beginners.

- **Seated Poses:** Seated poses can be uncomfortable at first, but they lead to improved flexibility and stability, helping the practitioner to open the body through posture awareness. In particular, the hips, chest, and shoulders benefit from seated postures. Common seated *āsanas* include *Daṇḍāsana* (Staff Pose), *Paścimottānāsana* (Seated Forward Fold), and *Sukhāsana* (Easy Pose).

- **Twisting Poses:** Twisting poses increase flexibility and core muscle strength. Depending on the twist, these poses also help to provide stimulation to specific organs. Twisting requires concentration on the breath. Common twisting *āsanas* include *Parivṛtta Utkaṭāsana* (Twisted Chair Pose), *Ardha Matsyendrāsana*, A (Half Lord of the Fishes, Version A), and *Sucirandhrāsana* (Eye of the Needle Pose).

Whether folding, twisting, or stretching, these maneuvers
are intended to elongate the spine, make space in the body,
and squeeze internal organs in such a way as to optimize
their functions.

*"By lessening the natural tendency for restlessness and by
meditating on the infinite, posture is mastered."*
-The Yoga Sūtra of Patāñjali, 2.47

At this point, it is important to note that practicing physical
postures supports holistic health, because above all, they
help to release stuck energy and move *prāṇa* throughout the
body. Everything is energy: the floor, the yoga mat, the
body, the breath, the thoughts, and everything in between.
Some energy moves faster than other energy (the breath vs.
the mat). Although we can't see it, the atoms that make up
the solid objects around us are moving, emitting their own
vibrational frequencies. Our bodies have a frequency, too.

As stated earlier, our bodies create chemicals that keep our
bodies working. Imbalances can cause issues but so can
stagnant energy. When we don't move our bodies, we don't
stimulate that energy. Maybe you sit at a desk all day long.
Maybe you commute for long periods of time. Or maybe,
you automatically go through the day without awareness of
how your body feels or moves. Sometimes, depression can

cause people to remain stagnant. When we don't move, the space in the body (vertebrae, joints, and organ tissue) becomes constricted, and any accumulated substances can get stuck, causing all sorts of ailments. Since emotions are literally chemical reactions in the body, repressed, unmoved, and unresolved emotions get stuck in the body, as well.

Energy that moves too fast can cause issues in the body, too. Anxiety, hyperactivity, and restlessness can cause the body to move too much, burning the body out and chronically keeping it on high alert. When we experience fear or nervousness, the body automatically transitions to the fight, flight, or freeze response. If you stay stuck in this mode, the body continues to emit epinephrine (adrenaline), norepinephrine, cortisol, and other substances. These chemicals are helpful in a panicked situation, but they are not good for everyday living. A regular *āsana* practice can help to relieve the symptoms of chronic stress and restlessness, which may lead to an overall calmer demeanor.

How to Effectively Build a Consistent *Āsana* Practice

"Practice becomes firmly grounded when well attended to for a long time, without break and in earnestness."
-The Yoga Sūtra of Patāñjali, 1.14

While many can feel the benefits of *āsana* after just one round on the mat, a regular practice established in regulated movement can help a person transcend *kleśas* (states of the mind, body, or spirit that cloud clarity and a calm heart-mind). Any ailment that obstructs optimal health and prevents you from achieving more peace (the intention of union) is a *kleśa* that can be removed. Awareness is the first step. The second is effort. It doesn't matter how long your practices are or what poses you use, as long as you maintain safety and regularity in your practice.

Set an intention (1-2 minutes): Intention is the foundation of yoga. An intention is a thought or words that move energy toward your goal. With "earnestness", you can work toward your goal during your yoga sessions, which then can continue throughout the day. Relieving stress, living in the present moment, or being more patient are simple examples that you can physically practice on the mat using breath and body movements. Your intention may change from day to day, but the overall method will provide you with an anchor to return to again and again.

Practice *Prāṇāyāma* (3-5 minutes): *Prāṇāyāma*, the fourth limb of *Aṣṭāṅga Yoga*, is the practice of controlling the breath. Breath awareness is essential to *āsana*, so the first step is to simply regulate the breath. Not only will this

99

regulated breath support your physical practice, but this short time period doubles as meditation.

- Sitting in *Sukhāsana* (Easy Pose), move your awareness toward your natural breathing pattern. Easy Pose can be as simple as sitting cross-legged.

- Begin to lengthen the breath, inhaling for 3 to 5 seconds and then exhaling for the same amount of time. This is a practice in retaining, slowing, and controlling the breath.

- Continue this practice into *Ujjayi Prāṇāyāma* (Victorious Breath). This breath is also called Ocean Breath, as it sounds like the ocean when practiced correctly.

  - Slowly inhale through the nose and then slowly exhale through the nose, making an aspirated sound ("ha"). Beginners may need to exhale through the mouth in order to get the throat to make the correct shape, which makes the correct sound.

- Use this rhythmic breath in tandem with your body's movements.

Begin *Āsana* (6-8 minutes): Again, *āsana* should consist of postures that move the spine in its six different ways; however, with enough practice, a practitioner can learn to customize his or her sequences based on intention and desired outcome (for example, *Sūrya Namaskār* (Sun Salutations) warm up the body, floor exercises can be grounding, and hip and chest openers can help release stuck emotions).

- From *Sukhāsana* (Easy Pose), move into *Bharmanāsana* (Table Top Pose). Here the practitioner moves onto his or her hands and knees, keeping even space between limbs and the spine straight.

- **Forward and Backward Spinal Movements**:

  - From *Bharmanāsana* (Table Top Pose), inhale while arching the back, bringing your belly toward the ground and tilting your chin/tail up (*Bitilāsana* or Cow Pose).

  - Exhale and move the spine in the opposite way, rounding the back and tilting the chin/tail down (*Marjariāsana* or Cat Pose). Repeat this pattern 5 times.

- Side to Side Spinal Movements:

  o From *Bharmanasanak* (Table Top Pose),
    return to *Sukhasana* (Easy Pose). Next,
    inhale slowly and raise the right hand
    toward the ceiling, bending the body toward
    the left. Keep your left hand on the mat,
    elbow bent slightly, while your right bicep
    stays near your right ear.

  o Exhale and return to *Sukhasana* (Easy Pose).
    Inhale slowly and raise the left hand toward
    the ceiling, bending the body toward the
    right. Keep your right hand on the mat,
    elbow bent slightly, while the left bicep stays
    near your left ear.

  o Exhale and return to *Sukhasana* (Easy Pose).
    Repeat this pattern 5 times.

- Twisting Spinal Movements:

  o In *Sukhāsana* (Easy Pose), make sure the
    spine is straight and that the hands gently
    rest on the knees. Prepare the body for
    Parivṛtta Sukhāsana (Simple Twist Pose).

- ○ Keeping an even breath, place your right hand slightly behind your right hip. Place the left hand on the right knee. Inhale and lengthen the spine.

- ○ Exhale and twist your body toward the right, looking over your right shoulder. It is important to move from your center/core. Take 3 to 5 breaths in this twist.

- ○ Inhale and return to center, placing your hands on their respective knees. Keeping an even breath, place your left hand behind your left hip, and place your right hand on your left knee. Inhale to lengthen the spine.

- ○ Exhale and twist to the left, looking over the left shoulder. Take 3 to 5 breaths in this twist.

- ○ Inhale and return to center. Repeat this cycle 5 times.

Transition into Meditation (2 minutes): *Śavāsana* (Corpse Pose) is an excellent way to end every *āsana* practice. It gives the body and mind a chance to cool down and process their exercise.

- From *Sukhāsana* (Easy Pose), lay the full length of the body onto the mat. Keep your palms up and a short distance from your sides. Point the toes outward and relax the feet.

- In this position, you can either lay quietly and in meditation, or you can scan the body, from toe to head, maintaining awareness of any aches or emotions you feel (released/stuck energy).

The above yoga sequence is an easy, seated sequence and is suitable for all levels. With practice, the body will become stronger (for stability and balance), lighter (for easier transitions), and cleaner (for a pure practice). Practice allows the body to continue onto more challenging poses, if desired, but an *āsana* routine need not be difficult to be effective. The important part is that you practice and devote your time to improving your body, mind, and spirit.

2

Prāṇāyāma: How to Maintain Health through Breath Awareness

"Calm is retained by the controlled exhalation or retention of the breath."
-The Yoga Sūtra of Patāñjali, 1.34

The brain and body cannot survive after three minutes of oxygen deprivation. Breathing oxygen is vital to our existence and the life force behind every living creature on planet Earth. But fueling our bodies with oxygen does more than keep us alive: Controlling the breath is the key to optimal health and wellness.

How does breathing and breath awareness impact our health? Many layers exist in this answer, but by living with breath awareness (and using the breath as a tool for wellness), you are supporting a healthy body, mind, and spirit. In Sanskrit, the word *prāna* means "breath" or "life force". According to yogic teachings, *prāṇa* sustains life and without it, an organism dies.

Physically:

- *Prāṇa* moves the energy of the body—blood, nerve impulses, lymph, etc.

- If we experience a disruption to our regular state (shock, stress, disease, etc.), that blockage creates irregular breathing patterns, which affect our physical state.

- With regular and controlled breathing, we can improve acute states of distress, as well as improve chronic dis-ease and maladaptive physical states.

Mentally:

- The mind will focus on the breath and go where breath leads, which aids in healing and meditation.

- Relaxation of the mind can alter gene expression, promoting physical and mental wellness.

- Breathwork and awareness is essential to *saṁyama*, the journey inward (inner limbs of yoga).

- Focus of breath helps yoga practitioners to reach *pratyāhāra*—sensory deprivation.

Emotionally/Spiritually:

- Breath or *prāṇa* helps to move energy and clear blockages in our subtle body—*marma* points (energy channels) and *cakras* (energy centers).

- *Prāṇāyāma* (regulation of breath) will calm the heart-mind and lead to inner peace.

By learning about the physical, mental, and emotional/spiritual benefits of breath awareness, you are working toward greater wholistic health and wellness. In regulating the breath and participating in breathing exercises, you can learn to use your life force to improve your health. This action is fundamental to yoga practice and positively affects all organisms.

What is Breath Awareness and How does It Impact Health?

To understand the importance of breath, in a yogic lifestyle, it is first important to understand the eight limbs of *Aṣṭāṅga Yoga*:

- *Yama* – abstinence

- *Niyama* – observance

- *Āsana* – pose

- *Prāṇāyāma* – control of the breath

- *Pratyāhāra* – sense withdrawal

- *Dhāraṇā* – concentration

- *Dhyāna* – meditation

- *Samādhi* – absorption

Breath awareness is the key to all limbs and at the root of all practice. For simplicity, this chapter will focus on *Āsana*, *Prāṇāyāma*, *Pratyāhāra*, *Dhāraṇā*, *Dhyāna*, and *Samādhi*. It is through practicing these limbs that one will nourish the body, mind, and spirit.

Breathing and Physical Health

Not only is breathing essential to living, but its quality is necessary to living well. First, let's deconstruct the physical anatomical actions during breathing:

- The diaphragm (a muscle just below the lungs) and the intercostal muscles (group of muscles between the rib bones) are responsible for your breathing, and they allow the lungs to function.

- Upon inhalation (breath in), the diaphragm and intercostal muscles contract and pull down and away from the lungs, which provide more room for the lungs to expand and fill with air.

- Upon exhalation (breath out), the diaphragm and intercostal muscles compress and curve into the lungs, which help the lungs to expel and push out the air.

Breathing is an automatic process. In the brain, the respiratory center located at the brainstem controls breathing. Mostly, the medulla is responsible for sending the message from the spinal cord to the respiratory muscles to breathe in and out. Further, the pons and other chemical responses in the body regulate breathing, involuntarily, by monitoring oxygen and carbon dioxide levels in the body.

Deep breathing increases oxygen levels and activates the parasympathetic nervous system (PNS). The PNS is the body's natural method of physiologically calming a person after the fight, flight, or freeze response:

- Regulates and decreases metabolism

- Decreases heart rate and blood pressure

- Increases nitric oxide levels (a vasodilator to expand blood vessels)

- Relaxes muscles

Physical Ailments Related to Breathing

When a person becomes stressed, frightened, or over-exerted (maybe through exercise), then the breath will shorten or even stop altogether. Have you ever noticed in a stressful situation that you were holding your breath? It isn't until the situation is over that you may realize this phenomenon. The body works in amazing ways to prepare you to respond and survive. When we are chronically stressed or living in a state of fear, however, it is possible to experience a host of physical symptoms and disease:

- Back, neck, side, shoulder, and chest pain

- Problems with blood pressure

- Sleep apnea

- Issues with hernias

- Stomach and digestive problems

- Wheezing, whistling sounds in chest

- Frequent headaches

These ailments can exist due to improper movements of the diaphragm and intercostal muscles, as well as increased carbon dioxide and decreased oxygen levels in the body. Shallow breathing and holding postures that chronically compress the body (slouching) can cause acute and accumulated physical problems. Unconscious breathing can lead to tight jaw, neck, and back muscles.

Women experiencing pregnancy may also notice that many of their symptoms are related to the breath. During pregnancy, normal breathing can become disrupted by hormonal changes (increase in progesterone) and physical changes (growing uterus, which impedes respiratory muscles). In addition, breathing is one of the key ingredients to enduring labor. Focusing on the breath, and keeping a consistent pattern, will help the mind and body through this extremely difficult process.

The most incredible aspect of breathing, however, is that although it is involuntary, it can also be controlled voluntarily! We demonstrate this ability to control breathing when we sing, speak, play musical instruments, or participate in controlled practices, such as *prāṇāyāma*. By controlling the breath, we not only work to calm the mind, but we calm the physical body as well. Deep breathing ensures adequate oxygen flow and the use of muscles involved in respiration.

Being aware of our physical posture and the status of our breath is vital to optimal physical health. People spend much of their time sitting at a desk, driving or riding in vehicles, and watching hand-held devices. These all corrupt good posture practices, which lead to poor breathing practices. Even people who exercise regularly may find that improper breathing patterns can hurt their bodies rather than aid in oxygen recovery.

Breathing and Yoga (*Āsana* and *Prāṇāyāma*)

The breath is the link between the physical and mental
activities, while practicing yoga and navigating everyday life.
During physical yoga practice (*āsana*), it is important to
link the breath to your movements, and to do so, it is
essential to focus on the breath and create a breathing
pattern. The best type of breathing during *āsana* is deep,
consistent inhalation through the nose while performing
expansive poses (chest openers, rising poses, etc.), and then
full exhalations through the nose (or mouth, depending)
while performing poses in which you fold into yourself
(downward movements, while twisting, etc.).

Note: The most important aspect of breathing to remember
while practicing physical postures is to keep breathing! Do
not hold the breath. Create a flow that becomes meditative
and helps to establish consistent breathing patterns you can
carry into future practices and daily life.

While *āsana* refers to the refinement of the body,
prāṇāyāma is the regulation of breath. Many classes exist
that focus on just *prāṇāyāma*. However, it is necessary to
also participate in breathing exercises on your own, which
will help you establish good breathing patterns. A guide to
breathing exercises exists at the end of this chapter.

Breathing and Mental Health

Taking deep breaths is one of the most common practices involved in stress relief and calming the mind. Parents use this technique with small children during tantrums. Medical professionals will guide their patients to use deep breaths during painful experiences. While deep breathing helps the physical body, it affects the mind in magnificent ways.

Calming the mind affects emotional states as well, which will be discussed later in this chapter. However, a calm mind is necessary in sustained and sharpened focus, diminishing the symptoms of anxiety and panic attacks, as well as reaching higher states of union (yoga) during meditative practices. But before we explore the benefits of breath awareness and mental health, it is important to understand how breathing affects the brain and mental states:

- Breath awareness can help you focus on the present moment, which can improve your attention span, diminish symptoms of anxiety, and boost overall personal awareness.

- Present moment awareness is also responsible for decreased mental fog and increased productivity (multitasking strains your mental bandwidth).

114

- Regular meditation can lead to positive changes in gene expression, naturally regulating blood pressure, metabolism, inflammation, sleep patterns, etc.

Training your brain to stop incessant mind chatter and to just Be is one of the most beneficial activities you can perform. A daily meditation practice, which includes focusing on the breath, is at the core of ideal health.

Breathing and Yoga (*Pratyāhāra* and *Dhāraṇā*)

On the path to wellness and union (*Samādhi* being the ultimate goal, which is union with the divine consciousness), it is necessary to train the body and mind. *Āsana* and *prāṇāyāma* help to refine the body and prepare the mind for meditation. Patāñjali does not spend much time focusing on physical practice, but *āsana* is intended to prepare the body for sitting comfortably in meditation. Once the body and breath are strong and consistent, a practitioner can begin to achieve *pratyāhāra* and *dhāraṇā*.

Pratyāhāra, or tuning out sensory input (sense control), is an important part of inner development. In "The Dawn of Light, letter 79", Hazur Maharaj Sawan Singh wrote, "The inner gate opens only when the outer gates are closed." This is an excellent analogy for understanding *pratyāhāra*. In

Sanskrit, *prati* means "against" and *ahara* means "that which is ingested". To clarify, *pratyāhāra* is the shifting from external distractions and attachment to internal focus and detachment. It is the bridge between the external and internal worlds, and it leads to many benefits:

- Helps to let go of attachments and stimuli that diminish peace

- Increases attention and focus

- Provides the practitioner more mental control (are you in control or is the external world?)

- Sharpens sensory input outside of meditation

When you can control and focus your attention (which is done through the breath), you purify the heart-mind, which allows light and love to enter without distortion.

Dhāraṇā is the first of the inner limbs of yoga and an integral aspect of meditation. In Sanskrit, *dhāraṇā* means "concentration". This fixed attention is the one focal point during meditation, such as an intention, object, person/relationship, or energy channels (any or all the *cakras*). *Dhāraṇā* is the first stage of *samyama*—turning inward—where the attention may wander and is called back to the focal point.

Breathing and Emotional/Spiritual Health

Regardless of how one looks at it, there is a subtle layer to the body that encompasses the way you feel. It is an exchange of energy; a situation is perceived, and we engage with the outcome in a positive or negative way. Some people believe that this subtle energy exists in centers and channels throughout the body, expressing themselves through *cakra* and marma points. This section will discuss these ideas, while supporting individuals who may only wish to refer to their emotional health without these references.

Meditation, deep breathing exercises, and breath awareness are methods used to purify the mind and control the emotions. As stated above, deep breathing can calm the body and mind, which can lead to an even emotional temperament. Think about when you are nervous, angry, or grieving. Taking a timeout to breathe deeply and to hush outside distractions is immensely beneficial to one's emotional wellbeing. But this practice, when continued down the yogic path, can also help to clear energy channels and maintain the health of the subtle body's energy centers. This practice allows *prāṇa* to move effortlessly throughout the body, which can lead to elevated emotional and spiritual experiences.

Breathing and Yoga (*Dhyāna* and *Samādhi*)

The breath is the single-most important aspect of turning inward to obtain emotional and spiritual wellness. Once you have used the breath to anchor your concentration in *āsana*, *prāṇāyāma*, *pratyāhāra*, and *dhāraṇā*, you will begin to unconsciously realize the benefits of single-pointed, continued focus. This consistent concentration is *dhyāna*, which is really continuous *dhāraṇā*. In this level, concentration is so focused that any external chatter (physical or mental) disappears, and you will be able to reach your goal. This type of meditation can bring clarity, inner peace, and move you toward *Samādhi*:

- Overcome deep emotional and mental triggers.

- Clear blockages that obstruct emotional healing.

- Clarify and stabilize your heart-center through consistent practice, which will carry over into your conscious awareness and everyday behaviors.

Since yoga means union, the objective of yoga practice is to clarify the physical body and heart-mind (mental and emotional states) to join with the divine, or higher Self. In other words, it is the goal to experience bliss, oneness, and absolute attention. *Samādhi* is complete absorption, the mastery of whatever our focal point is. When and if *Samādhi* occurs (after all, this takes practice and persistence), then you can begin to understand the object, person, or idea of your focus, without subjective judgments: Your knowledge has merged with the focal point and has become a part of your subconscious.

Using Breath Awareness for Everyday Health

Not everyone will master this level of meditation or yoga. However, in life, we can practice this sort of attention toward actions and objects by sharpening our concentration. We can do this while creating art, operating machinery, or even cleaning! When our minds wander, anchor back to the breath, and you help to create a pattern that literally changes your physical, mental, and emotional responses to the external world.

It is through this automatic process, one in which we take for granted, that we can improve every facet of our lives on Earth. Oxygen, *prāṇa*, is the force that moves through us all, and when we learn to harness it for health, we can live in harmony within ourselves.

Prāṇāyāma Practices:

There are several breathing practices that will help you to control, retain, and flow *prāṇa*. Here are two breathing exercises to practice anywhere:

Kuṁbhaka (Breath Retention):

In Sanskrit, *kumbha* means "pot" (the traditional image is of a human torso as a container for the breath with two "openings" at the throat and then at the base of the pelvis). Two types of retention exist: *antara* (internal) and *bahya* (outer).

Step 1: Sit in a comfortable, meditative posture. Ensure the spine is straight. Sit in a chair if necessary. Close the eyes and begin to breathe naturally through the nostrils.

Step 2: Now it is time for internal retention (*antara kuṁbhaka*). Take a deep breath and hold for five seconds (do this in your mind and use mala beads or fingers to aid your counting). Tuck the chin and place your thumb and ring finger on either side of your nose. This is called *mrigi mudra*, which means "deer seal". Hold the breath for five more seconds.

Step 3: Now it is time for outer retention (*bahya kumbhaka*). Release both the hand and head, tilting chin back into alignment, and fully exhale for 10 seconds.

Step 4: Repeat this pattern for 10-15 minutes. This exercise will help to improve breathing patterns, increase breath retention, and support the diaphragm and intercostal muscles.

Nāḍi Shodhana (Alternate Nostril Breathing):

In Sanskrit, *nāḍi* means "channel", and *shodhana* means "cleaning" or "purifying".

Step 1: Sit in a comfortable position or easy pose. Ensure the spine is straight. Sit in a chair if necessary. Make *mrigi mudra*.

Step 2: Close the right nostril with the thumb. Inhale through the left nostril, then close the left nostril with your ring finger. Release the thumb and open the right nostril, exhaling slowly out of the right nostril.

Step 3: Keeping the left nostril closed, inhale through the right nostril. Close the right nostril with the thumb, release the ring finger, and open up the left nostril. Exhale slowly out of the left nostril. This completes one cycle.

Step 4: Continue this exercise by performing three to five cycles. This exercise is intended to open the energy channels in the subtle body and balance oxygen levels to both sides of the brain.

3

Samyama: How to Travel the Meditative Path to Health and Wellness

"By the mastery of samyama, comes the light of knowledge."
The Yoga Sūtra of Patāñjali, 3.5

The health benefits of meditation are well known. Breathwork, mindfulness, and relaxation are all techniques used to destress, focus, and gain introspection. But meditation, according to the practice of yoga, is an essential step down the eight-limbed path.

The practice of meditation is a turning inward, a series of disciplined actions to realize a bounty of benefits. Consistent mediation has shown promising results, alleviating symptoms that plague the body and mind:

- Anxiety, fear, and stress

- Depression and low mood

- Post-traumatic stress disorder (PTSD)

- Obsessive-compulsive disorder (OCD) and other forms of incessant overthinking

- Attention- deficit/hyperactivity disorders (ADD/ADHD) and issues with focus

- Addictions and desires

- Dementia, memory loss, and aging

- Anger, resentment, and other difficulties with emotional regulation

- Problems with blood pressure, blood-sugar regulation/diabetes, and other organ system function

- Headaches and muscle tension

- Sleep issues and disorders

The list of symptoms and illness that meditation addresses is immeasurable. However, meditation doesn't just put the body, mind, and spirit back into alignment, it supports overall quality of life by enhancing mental clarity, physical performance, and spiritual enlightenment:

- Focus and attention to detail

- Creativity and inspiration

- Immune system optimization

- Vagus nerve function

- Gratitude, joy, and a sense of wellbeing

- Self-reflection and introspection

- Relationship with the Self and Divine Consciousness (God/Spirit)

- Hormonal balance

- Kindness, empathy, and connection

A consistent meditation practice can be life changing, but only one meditation session can prove beneficial. Most importantly, approaching meditation in a disciplined manner, will also lead to inner awareness. With *dhāraṇā* (concentration of the mind), *dhyāna* (continuous focus), and ultimately *Samādhi* (absolute attention), the last three limbs of the eight-limbed path of *Aṣṭāṅga Yoga* will lead to inner development and a heightened level of enlightenment.

What is *Saṁyama* and How Does It Lead to Inner Awareness?

To understand *saṁyama*, one must first know about the eight-limbed path of *Aṣṭāṅga Yoga*. As discussed in earlier chapters, the first four limbs consist of *Yama* (*ahiṁsā, satya, asteya, brahmacharya,* and *aparigrahā*), *Niyama* (*śauca, saṁtoṣa, tapas, svādhyāya,* and *Īśvara-praṇidhānā*), *Āsana,* and *Prāṇāyāma*. These are the principles and exercises to refine outer behaviors and personal practices. Beyond these are the practices that focus on inner development. These consist of *pratyāhāra* (tuning out sensory input), which is really the bridge between inner and outer control, then *dhāraṇā, dhyāna,* and *Samādhi*. While *saṁyama* translates to "focusing inward", it is comprised of the last three limbs:

- *Dhāraṇā*

- *Dhyāna*

- *Samādhi*

Meditation is the practice and execution of the last four limbs, culminating in "focusing inward".

Pratyāhāra (Sensory Withdrawal)

"Then follows supreme mastery over the senses."
-The Yoga Sūtra of Patañjali, 2.55

The last *sūtra* of the second book mentions the practice of *pratyāhāra*. The reason it is the last in book two is because its practice is considered to be the last of the outer limbs; however, its implementation leads to the inner journey. This action includes the external organs, which perceive stimuli. These are the ears, eyes, skin, tongue, and nose (at least). During meditation, the practitioner slowly begins to gain control of external input. This mastery becomes possible through *prāṇāyāma*, or breath control. By focusing on the breath, it becomes possible to diminish the importance and recognition of external sensory input. As Nicolai Bachman states, "The sensory organs now follow the heart-mind instead of the heart-mind catering to external sensory distractions" (p. 218).

Here, both Bachman and Śrī Svāmī Saccidānanda describe this mastery as driving horses. The horses are the sensory organs, the reins are the mind connected to the outer world, and the inner mind is the driver. Through breath work and direct focus (meditation), it is possible to become the driver, directing the outer mind. You can choose your focus, instead of allowing the world outside to choose it for you.

Dhāraṇā (Concentration)

"Dhāraṇā is the binding of the mind to one place, object, or idea."
-The Yoga Sūtra of Patañjali, 3.1

The third book within the *Yoga Sūtras* aptly begins with the practice of *dhāraṇā*. Even though it is not the first step in meditation (essentially the first five limbs prepare the practitioner for this moment), it is through choosing a direct focus that one begins to meditate. *Dhāraṇā* is the first stage in *saṁyama* and translates to "concentration." Essentially, this action is keeping the focus on one place.

For much of our awake life, we focus wherever our external sensory organs take us. Concentration requires filtering out that stimulation and directing your focus on one place, object, or idea. The place could be a vision in your mind. The object could be any tangible item. The idea could be any concept (keep it clarifying and uplifting).

The benefits of *dhāraṇā* are multifaceted and life-changing, because the ability to concentrate on one fixed point enhances the quality of the object of our attention.

Adversely, multitasking is a plague that diminishes the quality of a place, object, or idea. Lack of concentration leads to diminished outcomes, such as not fully relaxing during a vacation, not fully enjoying an activity (art, book, movie, song, etc.), producing sub-par results at work, and not being fully present in our relationships.

Not only does practicing *dhāraṇā* lead to further inner development, but it helps to sharpen everyday focus and attention. Choosing to focus on one item can calm the mind, diminish symptoms of anxiety (thinking of future) and depression (thinking of past), and allow you to harvest the necessary gifts of the present moment.

How to Practice *Dhāraṇā*

Although it is possible to practice with longer amounts of time and to focus on internal ideas, starting out with a five-minute concentration on a physical object is the simplest way to begin:

1. Pick an object to meditate upon. This could be an idea or vision, like the face of a loved one or the feeling you have when at your happy place, or you can choose a physical object. Good external objects can include a flower, flame, or religious symbol.

2. Sit in a comfortable position, either in a chair or on the floor. You may want to use a cushion. It is also possible to practice this lying down, but the intention is not to relax (or fall asleep), it is to actively concentrate.

3. Set a timer. It is suggested that beginners start with five minutes. It is important to start small, so you don't get discouraged. The depth of the practice is more important than the length.

4. Use the practices of *prāṇāyāma* to anchor the breath. Breathe deeply and rhythmically. The point of focus can be just the breath if you choose.

5. Concentrate on your chosen focal point. If focusing on an external object, keep the eyes open and the gaze relaxed. If focusing on an internal idea, close the eyes. When your attention drifts, simply bring your mind back to the point of focus.

It is important to note here that meditation should be a *sattvic* activity, intended to provide solutions, calm, and joy. If an object or thought disturbs your heart-mind, you may want to choose another focal point. It is possible to work out difficult issues or choices with meditation, but it takes practice and discipline of the mind to achieve this goal. The objective of *dhāraṇā* is to refine the mind (as *āsana* refines the body). Once the concentration is continuous, without breaking, the practitioner then reaches *dhyāna*.

Dhyāna (Meditation)

"Dhyāna is the continuous flow of cognition toward that object."
-The Yoga Sūtra of Patāñjali, 3.2

The second stage of *saṁyama* is achieved when no external stimuli distracts the meditation. *Dhyāna* is essentially a continuous flow of *dhāraṇā*. But what exactly is the difference, and how do we know when we've achieved this meditative flow?

In his translation of the *sūtras*, Śrī Svāmī Saccidānanda describes this continuous focus as getting lost in time. For example, if you sit and meditate for an hour, but it feels like only five minutes, then you have achieved *dhyāna*. If you meditate for five minutes, and it feels like an hour, you are still in the phases of *dhāraṇā*, or mere concentration. Other signs of *dhyāna* are feeling body-less, lightness, or warming sensations. Meditation experiences are personal and infinite. Accept what happens rather than enforcing your preconceived notions of what it should be.

In essence, *dhyāna* is the phase of meditation in which all else becomes mute, while the practitioner's stream of thought becomes fully merged with the focal point. The direct focus and concentration of *dhāraṇā* slowly begins to fade as you enter into a state of single-pointed focus. If during this phase, the practitioner's attention is diverted, becoming aware of external stimuli, then the meditation has gone from *dhyāna* to *dhāraṇā*. The shift among all three phases of *saṁyama* occurs often throughout meditation. Meditation is a practice, experiment, and journey into the Self, and there should be no expectations.

The benefits of *dhyāna* may be experienced at a deeper level than *dhāraṇā*. While the latter hones attention span and the ability to concentrate, *dhyāna* allows the heart-mind a moment to receive valuable insights and the energy of the focal point, which can purify and heal, without the constant chatter of the conscious mind. This monkey mind contains clouds—emotions and thoughts—which may obstruct the Self from Truth, Beauty, and Love. In yoga, these are the *saṁskāras*, or worldly impressions, upon the heart-mind. *Dhyāna* is a means to clarity, and clarity is a means to *dhyāna*.

How to Practice *Dhyāna*

To reach *dhyāna*, one must not break the flow of consciousness that occurs during *dhāraṇā*. *Dhyāna* occurs when concentration becomes uninterrupted, flowing continuously over the focal point. Bachman likens this to honey, flowing over the object, while *dhāraṇā* would be intermittent dripping of water onto the focal point. To achieve this phase, one must continue to practice *dhāraṇā* often and in greater lengths of time. It may become possible to slip into *dhyāna* more easily and quickly with continued practice.

Daily mindfulness exercises can also help the practitioner experience the benefits of *dhyāna*. While not sitting meditation, simple behaviors can lead to continued focus and blocking out external stimuli:

- Practice intentional listening during conversations, especially in noisy areas.

- Choose a difficult emotion, relationship, or circumstance and focus on that each day until you fully understand its essence.

133

- Shift your understanding of reality by seeing everything as a temporary Earthly version of consciousness. Look past the body, personality, and actions of a person to focus on the true nature that resides in us all.

These concepts may be difficult to understand without meditation practice, but the more you remove the temporary shell of what is perceived existence, then all that is left is Oneness. This complete absorption leads to the eighth and final limb: *Samādhi*.

Samādhi (Absorption)

"Samādhi is the same meditation when there is the shining of the object alone, as if devoid of form."
-The Yoga Sūtra of Patāñjali, 3.3

Samādhi is a complex concept, difficult to define and understand. Mostly, *Samādhi* must be experienced to comprehend its effects. It is not something that can be practiced. It is a destination and the last of the eight-limbed path. In Sanskrit, *Samādhi* means "absorption" or placing together. Its appearance, which occurs as the third phase of *samyama*, comes to the practitioner as complete contemplation. *Dhāraṇā* is directing the focus, *dhyāna* is

134

continuous flow of focus, and *Samādhi* is becoming the focus.

Imagine three points of existence: the point of origin (creator, God, the divine consciousness), the mind-body (the temporary vessels that are animate objects), and reality (the focal point of meditation, the present moment). The more the second point quiets and disappears, the better the chances that points one and three can meet. When the Source of life, the origin of consciousness, and the focal point meet, then you remove the temporary thoughts and emotions of the mind-body. This action reveals your true essence: You are consciousness—Awareness—experiencing itself with no boundaries. In this state, there isn't even a "you".

During *Samādhi*, the practitioner is unaware of this accomplishment, because that would denote acknowledgement and conscious thought. To achieve *Samādhi*, one must shift from awareness of one's self and the focal point, to an unconscious awareness of anything but the focal point. You are the focal point. The ego disappears. There is no "I".

Finding *Samādhi*

Samādhi is experienced when no sensory input is recognized, and the practitioner becomes completely absorbed internally. Remember, yoga is a journey toward union. There is no one way to reach this level of union, however, with consistent and elongated practice, the consciousness can find its way into the space of oneness on its own.

Going beyond the continuous focus of *dhyāna* takes time and practice; however, it is possible to reach *Samādhi* more easily as you become attuned to this enlightened state of being. You can practice meditation to obtain moments of *Samādhi*, but you can also catch glimpses of it throughout your day by becoming completely absorbed through an activity. *Samādhi* is the result of being wholly present in the moment:

- Get lost in a chore, exercise (try *āsana*!), or creative activity. Block out all sensory stimuli to fully focus on the task at hand. Zoning out without any other thought but the task is the desired outcome.

- Allow yourself to sit and do nothing. Be fully present in the moment. Do not pass judgments, do not evolve an opinion, do not entertain any perspectives. Simply be with all possibilities at once.

Consistent mediation can lead to healthy detachment, being able to observe rather than judge a situation as good or bad. This objective observation can lead to peace and a profound understanding of reality: The only moment is the present. Further, this inner journey can help the practitioner to release the ego. Everything is a embodiment of one, unifying consciousness, experiencing life through its various physical forms. There is freedom in releasing the temporary suffering of the mind-body, embracing the power of infinite awareness.

4

Nidra: How to Improve Your Sleep Quality to Enhance Health and Wellness

'Sleep is the mental habit characterized by the absence of form."
-The Yoga Sūtra of Patāñjali, 1.10

Sleep is an essential aspect of survival. During sleep, the mind and body recover from the previous day and prepare for the next. It is during this time that the body undergoes amazing processes that keep you healthy, safe, and happy:

- Cognitive functioning helps to process information to enhance memory and learning.

- Children and adolescents need sleep to develop according to their needs. Important hormones are released that ensure muscle growth and healthy puberty.

- Proper sleep allows the body to heal and repair itself. It is an important factor for immune function.

- Adequate sleep helps the body to regulate hormonal release that helps maintain a healthy weight and blood sugar levels. Sleep helps to prevent obesity and diabetes, and encourages healthy eating habits.

- A well-rested body and mind maintain physical and psychological safety. Sleep is an important aspect of performance.

Whether we have trouble with sleep or not (or think we don't), we could all improve our sleep quality. Sleep is an unconscious process, in which we are unaware participants. Yoga is the practice of focus and awareness. To live the yogic lifestyle is a calling to be more present and in control, even in sleep. Mastering the heart-mind through being more mindful about our sleep is a crucial step forward.

How Does Sleep Affect Your Health?

Sleep deprivation is the leading cause of many ailments, which include kidney and heart disease, diabetes, high blood pressure, stroke, depression, illness, and a range of chronic issues that can interfere with your daily life. Poor sleep patterns can also lead to mood issues and inept social interactions. More immediately, loss of sleep can lead to risks, such as auto accidents, poor work and academic performance, and other injuries.

So many times, we do not experience sound sleep. Receiving the necessary amount and quality of sleep is not as simple as closing your eyes. Many situations can interfere with a good nights' sleep:

- Anxiety or stressful thoughts can keep you from falling asleep and maintaining adequate sleep.

- Physical symptoms and illnesses, such as colds, allergies, pain, obesity, and pregnancy can make it difficult to experience healthy sleep.

- Sleeping at the wrong time of day can impede sleep cycles.

- Sleep disorders, such as sleep apnea, prevent you from experiencing all the sleep cycles that are necessary for rest and repair.

- Blue light (from computer, TV, and phone screens), diet or time of meal, and bedtime routine can impact healthy sleeping patterns.

Although you may believe that you achieve adequate amounts and types of sleep, the truth is that many of us are living with some level of sleep deprivation. It is recommended that adults sleep for at least seven to nine hours per night, and children and adolescents should be receiving up to at least 12 hours per night. But more important than quantity of sleep is the quality of sleep we receive.

The Importance of the Sleep Cycle

Good, quality sleep consists of experiencing the full cycle of sleep. Being able to participate in deep sleep levels helps to heal the body and allows the mind to process important information. Because of the many reasons people do not achieve deep sleep, many go through life literally starving for sleep (and often without realizing it).

Each night, the human brain should experience sleep that includes Non-Rapid Eye Movement (NREM) and Rapid Eye Movement (REM) stages of sleep.

Stage 1: A person experiences the lightest levels of "sleep" during this stage. Typically, we are still conscious and can awaken easily. It is during this time that the brain experiences alpha wave patterns (8 to 12 Hz), which exist during relaxed, present, and meditative thought processes.

141

Stage 2: NREM sleep technically starts during stage 2. Here the brain experiences theta wave patterns (3 to 8 Hz), in which the mind undergoes processes that help it integrate memory and learning. In stage 2, arousal rarely occurs, and we withdraw our senses. Subconscious thoughts, feelings, and intuitions can emerge during this time.

Stages 3 and 4: Stages 3 and 4 of sleep are the deepest NREM stages. Here, the brain experiences delta wave patterns (.5 to 3 Hz) that enable deep healing and restoration. While stage 4 is a deeper level of sleep than 3, they are both where the unconscious mind exists. It is extremely difficult to wake during this period.

Stage 5: REM sleep occurs during stage 5. The brain experiences brain wave patterns similar to that of wakefulness (typically beta, 12 to 38 Hz). It is during REM sleep that people dream, which can contribute to important information and emotion processing.

The Importance of Stabilizing the Mind through Deep Dream States

"Mental stability also comes from observing dream and deep sleep states."
-The Yoga Sūtra of Patāñjali, 1.38

Physically and psychologically, the body and mind need to experience all levels of sleep. To live according to yoga is to alter the ways in which we experience typical life. When we sleep and dream in sub- and unconscious ways, we allow any form of information, memory, or emotion to affect our heart-mind. We can experience nightmares or dreams that affect our wakefulness. Even in dreamless sleep, we are subject to the whims of the physical and psychological body. These impressions (*saṁskāras*), can cause us more harm than we realize.

According to the teachings of yoga, four levels of sleep exist:

- Wakefulness (which is really sleep if we are neglecting internal awareness)

- Dream Sleep (in which emotions and thoughts are unconsciously experienced)

- Deep Sleep (that includes involuntary processes in which the seer is not actively involved)

- Beyond (which is where the seer experiences absolute nothingness)

In all actions, the yogic practitioner attempts to make all mental action *sattvic*. In Sanskrit, *sattva* refers to "purity", and its application is to increase that which brings light and health, while discarding that which brings dis-ease. Sleep is also an action, and it can affect our bodies in profound ways. When we apply our focus on producing sleep that will bring purity to the heart-mind, we can improve the quality of our lives tremendously.

To live according to *Sūtra* 1.10, it is essential to control the senses by purposefully engaging with uplifting sensory experiences (sounds, smells, tastes, thoughts, etc.) and avoiding harmful activities (like over-sleeping, sleeping in an environment that negatively impacts sleep quality, and participating in mind chatter that does not bring *sattvic* results). This can be done through a number of purposeful activities, incorporated into evening and bedtime routines, and by participating in *Yoga Nidra* (see below).

When we practice and protect our sleep, we safeguard the heart-mind. It is not easy to alter habits, especially in regards to a purely unconscious way of being; however, with practice and commitment, it is possible to not only alter our sleep, but we can obtain mental stability through keen observation (*niyama*) of our sleep and dream states. Through this observation, we can determine our needs and take control of what we allow to affect our peace and *sattvic* experiences.

How to Take Control and Manage Sleep

The last limb of *Aṣṭāṅga Yoga* is *Samādhi*. It is in *Samādhi* that the participant experiences complete absorption, nothing. In this nothing, we can find bliss. *Samādhi* is a total surrender—complete attention and focus. Deep sleep is similar to *Samādhi*, but when we are in deep sleep, we experience the opposite of complete attention and focus. Our minds and bodies seem out of our control. Thoughts, emotions, and memories spray in all directions, and our body relaxes, tenses, and experiences paralysis according to its own terms. The goal is to attain more focus in our sleep so that hurtful experiences do not lead to harmful impressions on our mind, body, and spirit.

Since we live in a contemporary society, and it is extremely difficult to adopt a complete yogic lifestyle, it is important to take control where you can:

- Be mindful of your habits during the day that may lead to difficulty sleeping at night.

- Participate in an evening and bedtime routine that prepares you for quality sleep.

- Create an environment that is conducive to healing sleep.

- Incorporate yoga into your routines and regularly participate in *Yoga Nidra* (yogic sleep).

Learning about and participating in Ayurveda (the sister-science of yoga), can help you to live a lifestyle that is conducive with the habits described below.

Day Time Routine

Everything you do in life affects all other aspects. Painful experiences, emotions, and memories can create lasting impressions on your body and mind. These *saṁskāras* can affect your quality of sleep. The substances we consume during the day can also affect our ability to sleep. Exercise, screen time, and physical health can all contribute to sleep quality. Here are some tips for daytime activities that will help you enhance your sleep:

- Participate in a morning routine (*dinacharyā*) that supports hygiene and health.

- Limit or eliminate caffeine, nicotine, and alcohol.

- Drink plenty of unadulterated water.

- Eat three well-balanced meals (last meal between 6 and 7 p.m.).

- Exercise for at least 20 minutes per day (*āsana* counts). Enjoy cardio-focused aerobics a few times per week.

- Take periodic time outs during the day to relax, meditate, or do nothing.

Evening and Nighttime Routines

How you spend your evenings preparing for sleep and dream time is important. By being mindful of evening activities that support or hinder sleep quality, you can build a routine that makes you feel cozy and satisfied:

- Limit blue light interaction (smart phone, computer, and television). Give yourself two hours without them before bed.

- Take a warm bath or shower. You can also incorporate a self-massage with oil to make you feel relaxed and nourished.

- Eat a light meal for dinner and eat no later than 7 p.m. (or try to eat 2 hours before bed).

- Set a regular and decent bedtime. Try to be in bed by 10 p.m.

- Participate in activities that prepare you for sleep (*āsana*, aroma therapy, relaxing music, candles, or *Yoga Nidra*).

Here are a few poses (*āsana*) that can help with sleep, either in preparation or when it eludes you:

- *Hastapadasana* (Standing Forward Bend)

- *Marjariasana* (Cat Stretch)

- *Shishuasana* (Child Pose)

- *Baddha Konasana* (Butterfly or Bound-Angle Pose)

- *Viparita Karani* (Legs-Up-The-Wall Pose)

Bedroom Feng Shui

You don't have to be a feng shui master to understand and implement some basic principles regarding your sleeping space. By acting intentionally about your treasured sleep space, you can enhance the quality of your sleep and create room for more focused, yogic sleep.

- Place your bed in the center of the room and maintain balance (a table or lamp on each side).

- Avoid placing your bed near anything that will distract you (too close to a work desk, under a drafty window, or too close to the door).

- Remove electronics and exercise equipment from sight.

- Eliminate light, especially blue light, from your sleeping space.

- Use relaxing aromas to support sleep. Lavender, clary sage, peppermint, rose, and sandalwood are some options, and each person will be attracted to different smells. Use a diffuser and essential oils, or hang a plant/herb in your bedroom.

- Be mindful of clutter and colors. A clean space with warm colors can help induce relaxing sleep. Try light blues, greens, and purples.

What is Yoga Nidra?

To go further, into the Beyond, practitioners can participate in *Yoga Nidra*—a powerful type of yogic sleep that leaves one feeling refreshed, rejuvenated, and restored. *Yoga Nidra* is a level of sleep that typically cannot be realized. In regular sleep, a person understands that he or she has slept, but whatever transpires during sleep and dreams occurs in an unconscious way, which can limit the benefits intended by sleep. *Yoga Nidra* is a focused practice. It can promote deep healing, can prepare you for more intentional sleep, and can provide essential rest.

One 30-minute *Yoga Nidra* session can be the equivalent of two to four hours of normal sleep. You can either find a session offered near you, or you can practice it in the comfort of your own home with the use of guided sessions. *Yoga Nidra* is a deep state of relaxation that alters brain wave cycles. It is a practice that helps promote sleep but in a way that exposes the participant to single-pointed focus during sleep-like experiences. With continued practice, it is possible to turn these deep healing sessions into meditative methods to help enhance inner awareness. The practitioner can develop mental stability through awareness of the sleep state, but *Yoga Nidra* is also a great practice to promote sleepiness in preparation of normal sleep.

Stage 1: This level consists of relaxing the practitioner and guiding him or her into a meditative and focused sleep. Beta brain waves, experienced during wakefulness, slow down considerably.

Stage 2: This level consists of deep belly breathing, which helps to increase serotonin in the brain. At this stage, the brain wave patterns slow to alpha, theta, and delta, which are experienced during normal sleep.

Stage 3: During this stage, the brain increases in alpha wave activity. Alpha waves promote mindfulness, which aids in concentration, memory integration, and other prefrontal cortex executive functioning. Research also indicates that this activity helps to decrease symptoms of anxiety and depression.

Stage 4: The fourth and final stage of *Yoga Nidra* promotes consistent delta brain wave patterns. Because of the way in which the practitioner reaches this stage, he or she experiences this deep sleep while maintaining conscious awareness.

Yoga asks us to be more intentional about our sleep. Observing our deep sleep and dream states can lead to powerful insights about ourselves. In addition to the information above, we can use the power of intention to be more mindful of what thoughts and emotions flood our minds and bodies within the moments before sleep. Avoid negative thinking. Envision what you want to experience in your sleep and dreams. And most importantly, pay attention to your sleep and dream patterns for underlying issues that may need to be addressed.

Overall, sleep and dreams are important aspects of everyday health. By living intentionally, and using various methods to sleep intentionally, we can increase the quality of sleep we receive, supporting our health: physically, mentally, and spiritually.

5

Śauca: How Cleanliness Paves the Path to Holistic Health

"Moreover, one gains purity of sattva, cheerfulness of mind,
one-pointedness, master over the senses, and fitness for
Self-realization."
-The Yoga Sūtra of Patāñjali, 2.41

A clear relationship exists between cleanliness and health. Physical fitness, hygiene, mental clarity, and emotional regulation produce a powerful package that supports inner and outer health. It is through the valuable practice of yoga that one can begin to observe cleanliness in a way that acts to deeply purify the body, mind, and spirit.

When we choose to lead a cleaner life, we simplify it. When we simplify our lives, they become cleaner. Clean living consists of intentionally choosing products that go into, on, and around our bodies that align with the fundamental principles of *Yama and Niyama*. These first two limbs of *Aṣṭāṅga Yoga* consist of

- Non-violence (*Ahiṁsā*)

- Truthfulness (*Satya*)

- Non-stealing (*Asteya*)

- Conserving vital energy (*Brahmacharya*)

- Non-hoarding (*Aparigrahā*)

- Cleanliness (*Śauca*)

- Contentment and gratitude (*Saṁtoṣa*)

- Causing positive change (*Tapas*)

- Independent study (*Svādhyāya*)

- Humility and faith (*Īśvara-Praṇidhāna*)

Discussed earlier in this book, these limbs describe a process and practice that work to purify the body, mind, and spirit through dedication to behaviors that clarify the whole human. This chapter will now focus more intently on cleanliness, which can be observed and practiced through maintaining the following:

154

- Clean body: hygiene, diet, exercise

- Clean environment: home, community, planet

- Clean heart-mind: mental, emotion, and spiritual center

Through practicing yoga, especially the eight limbs of *Aṣṭāṅga Yoga*, it is possible to increase vitality and support health. Health and wellness attract positive experiences and radiate to the collective, just as water ripples throughout a pond. When you take responsibility to maintain a clear heart-mind-body, you increase joy and stamina in your own life, and shine like an example of pure white light to all those around you.

What is *Sattva* and How Does It Lead to Health?

As is a foundational principle in science, the principles of yoga recognize that all matter is composed of energy. In yoga, this energy substance from which all matter exists is *Prakṛiti*. *Prakṛiti* is the "nature" of all (often referred to as the proper noun "Nature"), and it is comprised of three essential "qualities or attributes" called *guṇas*. The three *guṇas* are

- *Rajas* (activity and restlessness): This quality is the state of attachment, passion, and change.

- *Tamas* (inertia and dullness): This quality is the state of heaviness, inactivity, and apathy.

- *Sattva* (purity and balance): This quality is the state of gratitude, harmony, and equanimity.

All three *guṇas* are present in us all, and all three are necessary in certain quantities and at certain times. However, it is *sattva* and *sattvic* activities that balance and protect the body, mind, and spirit from the harm that *rajas* and *tamas* can create. *Sattva* is Beauty, Truth, and Love. It is the gentle and pure essence of anything we put into, on, and around our Being.

Cleanliness is an aspect of *sattva*. It is in cleanliness that we can obtain "cheerfulness of mind, one-pointedness, mastery over the senses, and fitness for Self-realization" (*Sūtra* 2.41). Honest intention leads to honest action. Honest action is choosing *sattvic* activities, ingredients, and behaviors. This purity will support physical health through diet, exercise, and daily routines. This purity will support mental health through calmness, focus, and contentment. This purity will support emotional and spiritual health through relationship, purpose, and positivity.

The Benefits of Maintaining a Clean Body

The physical body is the first place to start when choosing a clean lifestyle. The body is a difficult machine to keep clean, as it naturally collects and produces undesirable substances. The skin ages, the muscles ache, and the other parts of the body are a daily reminder that ailments are a part of life. Even though maintenance of this earthly vehicle is not a guarantee for health, it is a pathway toward eliminating the ailments that plague the body. Physical cleanliness consists of good hygiene, diet, and fitness, and it increases longevity and performance.

How to Practice Good Hygiene

Hygiene is a method of maintaining health through cleanliness. Regarding the body, hygiene means washing hands when appropriate, bathing regularly, and performing other routines to keep all aspects of the body safe from germs. Germs—bacteria, viruses, and other microorganisms—can cause dis-ease (discomfort), illness, and odor. It is important to practice good hygiene through a daily routine.

Each morning, start with a hygienic routine, based on the principles of *Āyurveda:*

Mornings (*Dinacaryā*):

- Eliminate waste from the body (this can be a useful way to monitor health)

- Clean mouth, eyes, and nose.

  ○ Use tongue scraper (metal spoon works well, too)

  ○ Gargle with warm saltwater

  ○ Brush teeth

  ○ Oil pull or swish

  ○ Clean nose with neti pot

  ○ Wash eyes with eye cup

- Clean body

  ○ Start with self-massage (*abhyanga*)

○ Bathe in warm water (to match body temperature) by either a shower or bath

Throughout the day, maintain good hygiene by washing hands after being in public, after bathroom use, and before/after meals. Cover any sneezes and coughs. Wear clean, loose clothing. These practices, along with a clean diet and exercise will help enhance physical health.

How to Practice Clean Eating

The seat of physical health resides in the gut. How the body digests food is an indicator of health. Clean eating consists of being mindful of ingredients, sources, and personal tolerance. A well-balanced diet, composed of whole foods and *sattvic* qualities, eating regular meals, and maintaining the digestive fire is the best way to fuel the body.

Water:

- After completing your morning hygiene routine, drink a glass of room temperature water. Add lemon if desired.

- Drink plenty of water throughout the day, which will support elimination and organ function. Each person should drink a half ounce to one ounce per pound (body weight) per day. For example, if you weigh 130 pounds, it is recommended that you drink 65 to 130 ounces of water per day. That's approximately 8 to 16 glasses. That's between a half and a whole gallon!

- Drinking tea (non-caffeinated) is recommended. Many herbs support different functions, but above all, drinking tea helps to support digestion.

Food:

- Whole foods are best for a clean diet. This list includes choosing foods that are unprocessed, natural, and low in additives:

  o Vegetables and fruits

  o Whole grains

  o Legumes and beans

  o Lean meats (if not a vegetarian)

  o Oils, such as coconut, sesame, olive, and sunflower

160

- Eat foods from ethical sources. Dairy, meat (including fish), and eggs should come from sustainable sources and from environments that choose *ahimsa*.

- Eat seasonally and locally, choosing foods that grow naturally in your environment.

- Eat three consistent meals per day, with lunch being the largest, as it needs to fuel your energy throughout the remainder of the day. Consistent meals will help maintain regular digestion.

These are general suggestions. It is also important to understand your specific energy qualities (*dosha* and *Prakṛiti*), balancing your body according to its needs. *Vata, pitta,* and *kapha* are three attributes that each person has. The goal is to find balance through diet and activity. For more information, see the supplement at the end of this book: *What is Āyurveda and How Does It Work?*

How to Practice Cleanliness through Movement

Regular exercise is an important part of cleaning the body. One of the *niyamas* is *tapas*, which means "to burn or heat". Exercise is an excellent way to clean the body of impurities, while regulating organ function. It is also an amazing way to boost mental clarity and emotional contentment. *Āsana* is an excellent way to support every cell of the body. It is through meditative movement that we can clean the body, mind, and spirit.

It is important to consider your personal body needs when picking an exercise routine: Intensity, length of workout, and regularity of routine are dependent upon metabolism, present organ health, and body type. For example, people with a primarily *kapha* constitution will need more stimulating routines that keep energy movement high (HIIT workouts, cardio, and brisk walks). People with a primarily *vata* constitution will need a grounding and calming routine (restorative yoga, cycling, and dancing). People with a primarily *pitta* constitution will need a cooling routine that encourages their competitive natures (long distance sports, swimming, and outdoor activities). Below are general exercise suggestions to clean the body through movement:

Āsana:

- Begin the day with a gentle and warming routine. A few rounds of *Sūrya Namaskār* (Sun Salutations) are a great way to welcome the day and get the body moving.

- Incorporate poses that are intended to clean the body systems, such as

  - *Viparītakaraṇī* (Legs-up-the-Wall Pose) drains the lymphatic system and improves circulation.

  - *Parivṛtta Utkaṭāsana* (Twisted Chair Pose) helps to detox the body by "wringing" the internal organs and moving the spine.

  - *Marjaryasana-Bitilasana* (Cat-Cow Pose) aids digestion through intestinal massage and in supplying fresh blood to the body.

- End the day with a relaxing and restorative session that focuses the breath, while helping the brain and body process the day's activities.

Cardio:

- Aerobics that move the larger limbs of the body will help to increase heart rate, which improves respiratory and circulatory health.

- Incorporate 20 minutes of cardio-vascular supportive aerobics into each day. For some, this includes a brisk walk, making sure to move the arms. For others, it may include jumping jacks, mountain climbers, stair climbers, swimming, biking, and more. Make sure to know your own heart health and consult with a doctor for an appropriate and personal plan.

The Benefits of Maintaining a Clean Environment

It is not enough to keep the body clean if the environment in which the body lives is unclean. A clean environment includes home, community, and planet. You do not need to be obsessive or overly consumed with sanitation, but good hygiene extends to the environment. As all our actions ripple out into the pond of the collective, the cleanliness of our environment has a significant impact on our health:

- Floors, countertops, and other surfaces

- Digital devices, such as cell phones, tablets, and remotes

- Air conditioning and heating ducts

- Property/yard, playgrounds, parks, and other public places

- Refuse collection and containment

- Gardens, farms, and food sources

- Air and water quality

Everything in and around our homes can impact our health, including every environmental phenomenon existing on the planet. From the ingredients in our shampoo to the quality of trash collection in each community, every decision regarding cleanliness makes a difference.

How to Maintain a Clean Home

Keeping your home clean can seem arduous after working all day, taking care of children, or simply juggling all life's demands. But with a disciplined and regular routine, you can create a home that is worthy of housing your body and your loved ones.

Tip: Try to use natural products, such as vinegar, alcohol, and essential oils to clean. A few drops of lemon, tea tree, thyme, or oregano can provide the antibacterial and anti-viral components your surfaces need. Also, try and choose personal hygiene products (or make your own) that limit toxins in your environment and on your body. These include deodorants, shampoo, body wash, and even feminine hygiene products.

Daily:

- Wipe down electronics, including remotes

- Clean bathroom sinks and handles, as well as toilet handles and seats

- Disinfect tabletops and kitchen counters after cooking and eating

Weekly:

- Wipe down handles on appliances, doorknobs, and light switches

- Vacuum and lightly dust (open the windows to let that energy flow)

- Clean non-carpeted floors

- Spray down the bathtub and clean toilet

- Wash sheets and towels, using hot water and adding a cup of vinegar

- Disinfect lunch boxes, water bottles, and other bags

Monthly or Quarterly:

- Clean curtains, windows, and windowsills

- Wash coats, jackets, hats, gloves, etc.

- Clean out vents, air filters, and other devices that affect air quality

- Deep clean the inside of appliances

How to Maintain a Clean Community

While considering your own health and safety, treat your community as if it were your home. The health of that environment directly impacts you, as well as your family and friends. The public library, playgrounds and parks, trash services, schools, clinics, and grocery stores should be clean. While you do not have much control over these environments, you can do your part to maintain a clean environment, which will enhance the health of all:

- Pick up litter, dispose of your own trash

- Tie up garbage properly and put out on designated days

- Make sure to dispose of possible toxins appropriately: medicines, batteries, and electronics

- Clean up after pets

- Send disinfectant wipes and tissues to school

- Cover your coughs and sneezes

- Attend community and school board meetings if you are concerned

- Submit concerns to local businesses

How to Maintain a Clean Planet

The health of Earth impacts the health of her inhabitants. Our existence depends upon access to uncontaminated water and air. The pollutants that go into our bodies can significantly impact our health, causing irreparable damage and even death. How we care for Earth is how we care for ourselves. It may seem difficult to affect change on a global scale, but any action you take to keep the planet clean is a step toward progress:

- Limit your carbon footprint by...

  o Planting a garden and eating your harvest

  o Eat less meat, meat from sustainable sources, or no meat at all

  o Unplug devices from outlets when not in use

  o Eat and shop locally

  o Line dry clothing

  o Shop at thrift stores

  o Drive less, carpool, invest in an energy efficient car, take public transportation, or bike/walk when you can

  o Invest in energy efficient appliances

- ○ Divest from dirty energy sources and companies that negatively impact the environment

- ○ Invest in reusable items and divest from single use plastics

- Act and advocate by writing letters to government officials and to the local newspaper

- Plant trees

- Teach your children to care for Earth and spend time in her presence

The Benefits of Maintaining a Clean Heart-Mind

The heart-mind is a collective term for the mental, emotional, and spiritual center. The heart-mind is consciousness. It is the center of our intentions and how we relate to the world, ourselves, and our Source (whether for you that is the Universe, God, or another entity). When we have a clean heart-mind, we approach every action—from us or others—in a calm, clear, and balanced manner.

How to Maintain a Clean Heart-Mind

We acquire and maintain a clean heart-mind through honest, non-harmful, and loving intentions. All of the actions above will lead to decisive mental activity, compassionate emotional regulation, and inspiring relationships with the collective, including Source energy. You can also practice the following to purify the mental, emotional, and spiritual faculties involved in achieving cleanliness:

- Read substantial texts from reputable sources

- Pray and be grateful

- Breathe

- Align with worthy principles and divine inspiration

- Love unconditionally and forgive easily

- Practice introspection and work on personal growth

- Avoid violent, oppressive, and dishonest influences

Clean living is more than eating salads and using metal straws, although these are excellent choices. Clean living is about taking responsibility to filter *all* that comes into and around your body, while emitting clean energy back into the environment. All our actions affect the health of everyone and everything, which in turn, affects individual health. Through intention, discipline, and clear action, it is possible to achieve cleanliness, which of course, is akin to godliness.

III

The Yogic Lifestyle:
A Foundation
for Abundance

1

Kleśa: How to Eliminate Ego's Control and Cultivate an Identity that Attracts Abundance

"Ignorance, egoism, attachment, hatred, and clinging to the body life are the five obstacles."
-The Yoga Sūtra of Patāñjali, 2.3

The ego, defined by psychological theory, is the mediating factor between subconscious desires and conscious reality, and it is responsible for shaping a person's sense of self-worth. While the study of psychology has encouraged people to cultivate a healthy ego, the study of yoga is based on eliminating the ego and identifying with a higher reality: You are not your body, mind, or possessions, but rather an all-encompassing "Seer". Awareness, itself.

Many people struggle with this concept, especially in our modern world where we work, play, and interact as unique individuals. While it is important to navigate our responsibilities in the roles we manage, our created identities often interfere with our ability to establish joy and abundance. How we see ourselves—our name, possessions, skin color, health—is a construct of the mind. And the

174

stories we tell ourselves about this identity cloud our reality and control the course of life.

Through practicing yoga, you can learn how to hurdle the obstacles to abundance and happiness:

- Ignorance

- Ego

- Attachment

- Aversion

- Clinging to Life

These mental and emotional obstacles, or *kleśas*, work against our ability to grow. It is through these distorted identifications that we focus on lack, hold onto that which hurts us, and unfairly compare ourselves to others on their unique life paths. In yoga, you can clarify the heart-mind and build a life, even in this modern world, that leads to the flow of abundance.

What is Wealth and What Stands in the Way of Abundance?

The ancient wisdom of yoga provides practitioners with a guiding light toward freedom and joy. Freedom is obtained through clarity, removing the obstacles from our path and seeing through all the mud. This freedom leads to profound joy. One of the ways in which yoga helps us is by accepting what is and by eliminating qualitative labels, such as good or bad. It is in life's experiences that we flow. It is in the present moment that we live.

According to "The Yoga Sūtras of Patāñjali", ignorance, egoism, attachment, hatred, and clinging to bodily life are the five obstacles that impede anything we need. To survive on this planet, all people need wealth, whether it is in cash, assets, or skills. The reality is that we must "purchase" what we need, and we do so through bartering (trading skill or possession for currency) and money.

Each person will have a different interpretation of what wealth is. Some people may view abundance as having millions (or billions) of dollars, large mansions, expensive cars, and lots of people serving them. Others may see abundance as having enough wealth to keep their loved ones happy and healthy. It is a sliding scale, and everyone has their own judgements. Neither is correct nor incorrect. However, it will be impossible to meet your goals if you live with an identity that acts as an obstacle to and not a conductor of wealth.

Avidyā (Ignorance)

"Ignorance is regarding the impermanent as permanent, the impure as pure, the painful as pleasant, and the non-Self as the Self."
-The Yoga Sūtra of Patāñjali, 2.5

Ignorance, or *avidyā*, is a stumbling block to obtaining anything you want or need. If you don't know how or why to proceed, how will you know how to act? In Sanskrit, *avidyā* is the lack of *vidyā*, which is awareness. What is the antidote to *avidyā*? Becoming aware. In the *Yoga Sūtras*, Patañjali illuminates the dangers of *avidyā*. In his translation, Śrī Svāmī Saccidānanda provides an example where a man sees a snake in the night. The neighbors are roused from their sleep, one shining a light on the animal. But it is not a snake, it is a coiled rope. In our ever-busy, ever-noisy world, we too can make assumptions and misperceptions about reality. It is through the practice of yoga that we can shine a light on the darkness that clouds our judgment.

Avidyā can hinder many facets of our lives. Pertaining to wealth and abundance, it can keep us stuck in negative patterns. This lack of awareness can inhibit your ability to make decisions that help you accumulate wealth:

- Losing money to hidden fees or high interest rates

- Neglecting investment opportunities

- Not knowing about savings plans that offer a higher yield

- Not using consolidation and other tools to eliminate debt

Ignorance of financial tools and alternative methods (than what you currently use) can make you lose money and opportunities to grow your assets. Fear of change and lack of motivation prevent people from researching and implementing strategies for financial health. Even if you don't think you have choices (living paycheck to paycheck, having significant debt, or lacking time), you do. Plenty of tools exist online and in books (go to the library!). This information is free. Even if you save a dollar a week, transfer credit card debt to an interest free account, or put your savings in a high-interest account, you are acting. You are shining a light on your snake in the dark.

Asmitā (Egoism)

"Egoism is the identification, as it were, of the power of the Seer (Puruṣa) with that of the instrument of seeing [body-mind]."
-The Yoga Sūtra of Patañjali, 2.6

In Sanskrit, *asmitā* means "I am-ness". In the practice of yoga, identifying with the "I" and all its earthly aspects leads one to a distorted sense of self. Our view of ourselves becomes distorted when we identify our being with that of the physical body, our emotional states, the thoughts of the mind, our role in society (occupation and socio-economic class), and our possessions. Through the practice of yoga, the practitioner begins to understand that we are not these things. They are but an outer experience. Our true being resides inside. We are Awareness itself. We are the Seer.

Yoga Sūtra 1.3 explains this concept a bit further: "Then the Seer (Self) abides in Its own nature." The ego is of this world, and it is always changing; the Seer/Self is never changing and is the true essence. Imagine that your face is this Seer. If you look in a dirty, cracked, or colored mirror, your face changes. If you look in a clean, clear, and pure mirror, you can see your face for what it is. Yoga clears our vision. It removes the filter of the worlds' obstacles. When you begin to see yourself as a part of all the universe—no better, no worse than any other being—you see yourself as you are. You are not your car, your house, your job, your health, your emotions, or your thoughts. You are the pure light of Awareness.

The ego is concerned with these things. It is concerned with comparisons. It can create havoc in your life, which can affect your financial security:

- Nothing is good enough, and so you are ungrateful and wasteful.

- You will do anything to be right or win, even to your detriment.

- You feel insecure and anxious, which makes you either frozen in your approaches to finances or erratic in your decision making.

- You are too serious and overly concerned with titles and how other people see you, which can make you perform according to the ego's will.

- Being condescending or treating others with derision closes you off to opportunities and relationships that can improve your circumstances.

When the ego grows, it controls the life. It can make people corrupt from power. It can make individuals look down on others. It can cause people to try and harm others to "win" at all costs. Deep down, *asmitā*, is rooted in fear and insecurity. It is holding tightly to power, success, and material wealth, not for the good of others but for others to see. Humility, contentment, and gratitude are the ways out of ego-driven choices. When we work to remove our blemishes and improve ourselves—in a sincere and heart-centered manner—then we can make decisions that support authentic growth.

Rāga (Attachment) and *Dveṣa* (Aversion)

> *Attachment is that which follows identification with pleasurable experiences."*
> *-The Yoga Sūtra of Patāñjali, 2.7*

When we experience something good, like a raise or bonus, we experience temporary pleasure. While these events are nice, attachment to the feelings they give can sour your future expectations. Here, you can let your emotions and desires affect your work or the benefits you receive. This same principle applies to investments and other financial decisions. Sometimes, we can become emotionally attached to a particular company, stock, or bank. *But I've always banked with....* or *I believe in what this company stands for...* are examples of how we can let our emotional attachments determine our financial health.

While loyalty and investment in benign companies (and divesting from malign ones) is important, it is harmful to continue to invest in a company, bank, or other institution that no longer serves your needs. Companies change and so do their benefits. By not reviewing, re-evaluating, and changing in accordance with your present needs, you are harming your financial health.

Aversion is that which follows identification with painful experiences."
-The Yoga Sūtra of Patañjali, 2.8

In the same way, aversion, or *dveṣa*, can cloud your judgment. Just as we strive for pleasurable experiences, we avoid painful ones. These painful experiences, and the emotions we attach to them, determine our path. When we experience a financial defeat through unemployment, demotion, or investment loss, we can allow that defeat to deter abundance.

Below are examples of how attachment and aversion can influence your financial health:

- You continue to lose savings because of high bank fees, because you are scared to change banks.

- You don't apply for the job you want, because you are afraid of failure due to past experiences with employment.

- You stay in the same job, even though it is detrimental to your mental, physical, or financial health.

- You remove money from investments for fear of loss, before they have time to mature. The key to investment wealth is longevity.

- You have lost wealth in the past due to investments, and so you refuse to take part in sound and beneficial financial decisions.

- You become addicted to gambling or gaining wealth through risky behavior, which causes you to lose financial stability and the motivation to earn income through more reliable resources.

Attachments and aversions to circumstances alter behavior. Yoga requires that we let go of this "coloring" (the meaning of *rāga*) and view life's circumstances through a clear heart-mind. By removing these emotional triggers, we can be rational and judicious with how we approach financial decisions.

Abhinivesa (Clinging to Life)

> *"Clinging to life, flowing by its own potency [due to past experiences], exists even in the wise."*
> -The Yoga Sūtra of Patāñjali, 2.9

Clinging to life is fearing death. Death changes life (and life changes death). Fear is an instinct that humans have. This fear inhibits people from living authentically and inhibits them from taking necessary risks. This concept is akin to *dveṣa* (aversion) in that the fear of loss prevents us from acting in ways that attract what we need.

Abhinivesa is an obstacle to attracting abundance, because it makes people choose from a place of alarm and hysteria. For example, think about all the things you can insure: your health, house, car, animals, property, business and employment, and in some cases, a part of your body involved in your profession. You can even insure your life.

While it is important to make sure that the loss of anything (including your life) will be recuperated, these decisions must not be made in haste. With proper research (removing *avidyā,*) and rational decision making (removing *asmitā, rāga,* and *dveṣa*), you will learn to make investments for the long term that are not rooted in fear.

This clinging can make us blind to the beliefs we adopt. We will participate in social norms that may not make sense for our individual and familial needs. For example, a fear of death can easily make a person buy unnecessary products that promise longevity, when in fact, low stress, proper diet, and consistent exercise are the keys to health (try yoga!). In the same way, it may be more prudent for you and your family to purchase less life insurance and invest in other methods that will bring you more wealth. In the end, you must not get caught up in quick fixes and work toward creating abundance in a real and lasting way.

The Authentic You and Abundance

The most important takeaway of understanding the *kleśas* (obstacles) described by Patāñjali is that everything—except for the ever-present, constant Awareness—changes. Knowledge and information change. Your body, mind, emotions, and material possessions change. Circumstances

185

that bring you pleasure and pain change. Death of this body comes to us all, and so life changes. It is important to remove any ignorance, egoism, attachment, aversion, and clinging to this life. These are not who you are. To practice yoga is to move toward union. When we forge our identity as a *Being* that is a part of the whole, when we align our *Being* with the *Being* of all. We achieve union.

To accomplish these purities, one must participate in a consistent yoga practice. Self-inquiry and examination are a part of becoming the Seer. In "The Yoga Sūtras of Patāñjali", Śrī Svāmī Saccidānanda describes practice as a habit:

> When we do something several times, it forms a habit. Continue with that habit for a long time, and it becomes our character. Continue with that character and eventually, perhaps in another life, it comes up as instinct. (87)

2

Satya: How Authenticity Leads to Attracting Abundance

"To one established in truthfulness, actions and their results become subservient."
-The Yoga Sūtra of Patāñjali, 2.36

The path to wealth isn't always clear. But attracting what you desire, what you really want for yourself, is a direct journey. By identifying your goals and living in truth, you can find a way to what wealth you seek.

To live an authentic life means to live in absolute honesty. It means to speak, think, and act with clear intentions. Not only is this beneficial for others, by means of a reliable example, but it is essential to be true to oneself when pursuing dreams. Each person has unique gifts, intelligences, and methodologies. Humans differ in experiences and abilities, because the collective needs these varying perspectives and talents to create a wholistic system that sustains life on this planet. When we all choose to live an authentic life, according to our abilities, we give and receive what is needed, living in balance.

Leading from a clear heart-mind attracts abundance in many areas of life, because it allows individuals to reach their goals in the following ways:

- Setting honest intentions and following through leads to goal achievement.

- Using clear and direct communication provides according to expectations.

- Being honest and acting according to one's word will lead to trustworthiness.

- Authenticity means living in the present, which limits symptoms of depression or anxiety.

- Expressing emotions helps to regulate body systems, keeping channels open and life-force energy (*prāṇa*) flowing.

Authenticity is the mark of a responsible person, but it is also the means to finding purpose and joy. The practice of yoga is multilayered, and the effects are not always predictable. However, the practice of *satya*—living in truth— maintains alignment with intended goals and desires, attracting abundance in its many forms.

What is *Satya* and How Does It Lead the Way to Wealth

Satya is the practice of honesty. As the second *yama*, *satya* is a powerful commitment to the truth. Its practice is fundamental to the yogic lifestyle; one cannot attempt to approach the path to clarity without truth at its base. A healthy body depends on honest and clean behaviors. A healthy mind depends on dedication to the truth and filtering out falsehoods. A healthy emotional center depends on clear intentions and honest actions that lead to wellness. A healthy spiritual practice consists of the search for truth, without dogma or zealotry, continuously seeking and recognizing the divine in everything.

When these components are put together, they create a solid core, supportive and open. An honest foundation is capable of identifying the illuminated path forward, content on working in the present to meet the goals of the future. This active living in truth is particularly advantageous in regard to financial goals and building the wealth one desires. Disclaimer: The advice within these pages cannot make you rich. Not only is that delusional (a muddy filter from which we see the world), but it is against the tenets of yoga to describe this sacred practice to make money. However, with deliberate action, focus, and honesty (tenets of yoga), it is possible to fulfill intentions, carving a path toward financial freedom.

Authentic Intention

To begin down the path of creating your own reality, it is essential to understand the power of intention. Intention is a plan, goal, or objective. An intention can be general or specific. It can be a small goal or a large plan. Examples of financial intentions include:

- Spending less money

- Paying off debt

- Saving more money

- Growing investments or retirement savings

- Purchasing something specific

- Increasing generosity and charitable giving

- Starting a new business

- Moving to another location

- Carving a new life path

Each one of these goals can further be dissected into smaller actions. For example, spending less money may include investing in a coffee maker and reusable mug, instead of buying coffee every morning. A change as large as moving to another location will require research, travel, and making a financial plan (which then includes employment, cost of living adjustment, buying/selling a home, etc.). And then, each of these steps include smaller steps still. Regardless, once you set an intention and act to follow through, you will be amazed at how circumstances begin to fall into place. The important factor is to be authentic when setting intentions, being honest about desires and circumstances.

Being authentic about intentions means you must set goals that are in alignment with high-energy frequencies, such as Love, Beauty, and Truth. In terms of yoga, this means that you must set intentions and then act in a way that aligns with the principles inherent within the practice. These include the *yamas*, *niyamas*, and all other actions involved in creating a clear heart-mind.

For purposes of improving finances and creating wealth, it is important to set an intention that is honest. Stealing, cheating, or hoarding are not the ways to wealth. Neither is dreaming of a life that does not fit in with your purpose or abilities. It is impossible to desire wealth and then sit at home hoping it will magically come to you. You must determine what your financial goals are, in an honest way, and then move to act.

How to Set Intentions

Intentions become reality, so it is important to set ones that you really want to manifest. *I intend to become rich* is not a realistic objective. However, *I intend to align with my purpose/talents* or more specifically, *I intend to earn a certificate to bolster my education and credentials* are more in alignment with authenticity.

- Take an honest inventory of your financial situation. Make a spreadsheet or use an online tool to determine your net worth. Net worth includes assets (what you own) and liabilities (what you owe). Subtract liabilities from assets to determine your net worth.

- Analyze your spending. List all expenses and keep track of spending. Do you spend more than your paycheck? Cut spending. If you have something left over, invest.

- Make a list of short-term and long-term financial goals. Do you want to spend less money at the grocery store? Do you want to be debt free in three years? Do you want to change professions or grow your business? Then determine specific steps to reach these goals.

Once you have taken an authentic look into your financial situation, you can determine your intentions. Where do you need to flow your monetary energy? How can you accomplish this goal? Do you need to spend more, earn more, save more, or invest more? Regardless of your personal goals, understanding one's personal financial situation is the first step toward setting authentic intentions.

Authentic Communication

Communication is an essential part of reaching one's goals. Thoughts and words become reality. These are intentions. Honest communication leads to positive results. Even if you experience setbacks or difficult situations, taking authentic action will lead to achieving goals. However, authentic action cannot exist without authentic communication.

Authentic communication consists of honest language that we tell ourselves and others. The intentions above start as thoughts (communication with the Self). These words then become mantras, spoken aloud to oneself and then to surrounding people. This communication can be with an employer, friend, partner (business or romantic), or even a stranger. You are also a witness to your communication.

Intentions are not the only time we need to use authentic communication, however. Meaningful relationships depend upon honest communication. People must be able to trust the words you speak. They must see that not only do you speak in clear terms, but you also execute (authentic action) according to your conversations.

How to Practice Clear Communication

It's important to practice honesty in all communications in order to meet one's goals. Whether these are personal financial ambitions or maintaining relationships, authentic communication is the key to success.

- Don't mask a financial situation. If you cannot afford an activity with friends, be honest. Overspending will thwart your financial plans and resentment can become an issue in relationships.

194

- Be honest in business dealings. The more partners, employers, or employees trust you, the more opportunities will manifest.

- Clear communication will lead to the results you want. Be explicit in your language when making requests. You cannot expect to receive what you desire if you cannot clearly ask for what you need.

Practicing *satya* in communication is an essential part of living a yogic lifestyle and meeting financial goals. Authentic intentions lead to clear communication, which leads to authentic actions (communication is also a form of action).

Authentic Action

Honest action starts with honest communication (thoughts and written/spoken words), but it extends to the measures one takes to reach a goal. An intention may consist of paying off debt. Communication may consist of writing-in a line item to your budget to pay off a specific debt. However, if this is as far as you get, then you are not taking authentic action. Acting honestly in this situation means following through and carrying the energy of your intention forward. Walking the walk—executing your goals—is the most essential ingredient when meeting your goals.

How to Practice Honest Action

- Use tools to help you act according to your intentions. Calendar reminders, clock alarms, online spreadsheets, financial websites and apps, and other tangible instruments can provide the support you need to act.

- Act on your to-do list. After you've transferred your intentions into communication (a list), dissect the parts into action items. If you pledge to give more to charity, write that check today. If you pledge to grow your business, open a new bank account, clear out a space in your home for an office, or build your new website.

Authentic action is noticeable. Not only will others trust you more if you act reliably, but you will continue to move the energy of your intentions forward, leading to physical results and more opportunities.

Authentic Living

Authentic living is an intention in and of itself. Setting realistic intentions, communicating one's goals, and then taking authentic action leads to honest living. Authentic

196

living is habit forming. Annie Dillard said it best in "The Writing Life":

> How we spend our days is, of course, how
> we spend our lives. What we do with this
> hour, and that one, is what we are doing. A
> schedule defends from chaos and whim. It is
> a net for catching days. It is a scaffolding on
> which a worker can stand and labor with
> both hands at sections of time. A schedule is
> a mock-up of reason and order—willed,
> faked, and so brought into being; it is a
> peace and a haven set into the wreck of time;
> it is a lifeboat on which you find yourself,
> decades later, still living.

The power of authentic living becomes apparent with the results. Śrī Svāmī Saccidānanda explains this when he discusses *Sūtra* 2.36. When the yogi practices *satya*, in all facets of living, outcomes become a byproduct. The more one practices honesty, even if that honesty is a curse, the more he or she will see the results come true.

Authentic living also consists of living in the present moment. It is true that if you want to achieve goals, you must plan for the future, but action (and living) can only occur in the present. Both past actions and future ideas are constructs of the mind. They are also aspects of time we cannot control. By living honestly, right now, you can work to move the goalposts forward. Present living may also help to alleviate any feelings of regret, depression, or anxiety.

How to Live Authentically

In terms of finances, living authentically means being disciplined. It means identifying your principles and committing to them. This commitment may consist of the following:

- Buying locally, from small businesses rather than from online corporations, to support your community, balance power, and limit your carbon footprint

- Participating in second-hand exchange opportunities to limit the waste of production

- Making or fixing material goods rather than purchasing them to save money

- Investing in clean energy sources and divesting from systems that harm people, animals, and the planet

Ethical financial decisions ripple out, affecting everything. When each person decides to make more prudent and honest choices regarding how they use their money, the power shifts to honorable outcomes.

Authentic Expression

Authentic expression is more than honest communication and movement. It is the ability to identify and relay emotional responses in any situation. The ability to express one's feelings and reactions is not easy: Many people choose to repress anger, sadness, and other emotions (even joy and elation), because often, it is easier to avoid such vulnerability. Expressing emotions can challenge relationships, personal or business, but this honest approach helps keep communication clear and the energy within your body moving. Moving emotional energy is essential to prevent injury and dis-ease.

How to Practice Authentic Expression

It may be difficult to separate personal feelings from financial situations, but they are highly informative to the process. Here is how to use your emotions to guide you, making wise economic decisions, while maintaining health and wellness:

- Listen to your instincts. If something feels bad, most likely it is. Do not confuse types of anxiety. Nervousness exists to keep your mind in check. Re-evaluate your choices, and if they make you excited, go for it. If they make you upset, hold off.

- Openly communicate how you feel with everyone you work with. If someone's actions upset you, pause and reflect. Are your feelings valid? Most likely they are, because you are feeling them. Tell the other person as directly as possible how you feel (and possibly what would make you feel better).

- Readily share your ideas. Your idea could improve efficiencies, profits, or completely innovate the industry. Your ideas are a gift to the world.

Authenticity is a lifestyle. Honest intention, communication, action, living, and expression is a wholistic path that can do no harm (*ahiṃsā*). Clear thoughts and words become clear expectations, which will lead to desired results. It is possible to reach any goal, but it must be in alignment with truth, and that truth must be applied to every facet of one's life path.

3

Asteya: How to Practice Non-Stealing to Attract Wealth and Abundance

"To one established in non-stealing, all wealth comes."
The Yoga Sūtra of Patāñjali, 2.37

Stealing seems like a simple act. A person takes possession of an object that belongs to someone else, either by force or through cunning, Theft and robbery affect the collective economy and individual victims, leaving behind loss, mistrust, and trauma. But stealing doesn't have to be outright and obvious to affect both victim and culprit. Stealing includes many more actions, little dishonest behaviors that not only hurt others but negatively impact your ability to attract wealth.

Most often, we are not aware of our thievery. Common and unconscious theft can include the following:

- Running an errand or taking a break on company time

- Taking office supplies for personal use

- Consistently being late for meetings and events

- Keeping an object that you find, rather than find its owner

- Taking advantage of someone else's generosity

- Maintaining attachments to unused items

These are simple situations that range from serious issues to what seem like benign behaviors; however, when we steal time and resources, we not only hurt others, but we block the flow of abundance coming to ourselves. And stealing can take other forms, forms that don't necessarily have to do with time and materials. Anytime we rob ourselves and others of joy, peace, or safety, we are also stealing.

There are many ways in which we take. By practicing yoga, we can become more aware of our own actions and work toward non-stealing behaviors in all we do. This step can lead to a clearer heart-mind and can open us up toward giving and receiving in ways the unconscious mind has never imagined.

What is *Asteya* and How Can We Practice It?

As stated in a previous chapter, *asteya* is the third *yama* (restraint) in the eight limbs of *Aṣṭāṅga Yoga*. Again, the *yamas* consist of non-violence (*ahiṁsā*), truthfulness (*satya*), non-stealing (*asteya*), conservation of energy (*brahmacharya*), and non-hoarding (*aparigrahā*). These practices are the pinnacle of preparing one's heart, mind, and spirit to live a "cleaner" life and finding one's way toward ultimate unity (the purpose of yoga).

In Sanskrit, *asteya* refers to the act of "non-stealing." This *yama* considers all actions—thought, word, and deed—that involve theft. Every day, we act in ways that deprive others and ourselves. Every action elicits a reaction, whether the theft leads to legal trouble, mistrust, or limiting means and opportunities for wealth.

If caught, stealing can lead to legal troubles, which are costly and time consuming. You can lose your job. You can have a difficult time finding future work. You can pay thousands of dollars in fines and lawyers' fees. You can go to jail. If your behavior goes unchecked, it can still have powerful ramifications on your ability to accumulate wealth. When you limit others around you, you steal from yourself. Fewer resources for others leads to their own desperation. What they don't have, they can't give. In the same way, giving lends to more giving.

Money and Material Resources as Energy

First, it is important to understand that everything is energy, and this includes money and material objects. For abundance to flow to you, however you define it, you must be an open and reciprocal vessel for this energy. When we live in a state of mind that takes with malign intentions, we restrict the flow of benign blessings to us. Here are some examples of how hurting others through stealing negatively impacts our ability to attract wealth:

- When we steal time from an employer, we limit their productivity, which in turn cuts into their profit. If they do not make a profit, they cannot share their wealth with you.

- When we take supplies from an employer without repayment, they again lose money. This lost money cannot find its way into your paycheck.

- When we are continuously late for events, we can miss out on valuable information, and chance meetings and opportunities. We may even lose respect, being unreliable.

- If we find an object and keep it as our own, we are limiting the generosity of the original owner (think rewards and gratitude). We cannot expect people to return our lost possessions if we do not honor other people's property.

- If someone lets you borrow an item, takes care of you in any way, or provides you with a valuable service, it is good to accept that gift. But if you allow that person to consistently do so without reciprocity, you can diminish their spirit of generosity and their resources.

- If you keep an object beyond your use for it, you keep it from other people. By clinging to such items, you steal space from yourself, create an unhealthy emotional attachment to temporary material, and prevent others in need from harvesting the benefits of these resources.

Now, it is equally important to remember that each of us are only able to give what we have. Reciprocation is not a matter of "even" exchange (which can devalue giving), but it is a matter of recognition and sharing our individual gifts when they are needed. Stealing time and resources, and focusing on taking without giving, creates a stagnant flow of energy. In this stuck energy, we find ourselves feeling deprived, even if we are the beneficiaries. Why do people take without thoughts of giving? Because they feel as if they lack something. They may take out of revenge, fear, or desperation. Regardless of the reason, this action only serves to deplete.

In the opposite way, giving opens the channel for this energy to flow back to us. Shifting our minds from fear, desperation, and revenge will allow us to act in a way that puts us in alignment with more opportunity:

- Clocking out during your personal breaks and using your employers' supplies for their intended purposes will help keep their business in order. This benefit can provide profit for them, which they can then share with you (keeping you employed or providing a raise/bonus). You may also be an employee with integrity, which can put you in a better position in the company.

- Being on time can mean that you are where you are supposed to be. This can open you up to important conversations and events that lead you to beneficial circumstances.

- By being honest with other people's possessions, you open yourself up to trust. When people trust you, they can provide further opportunities to you.

- By supporting people's giving by reciprocating in your own unique way, you leave the channel open to receive more. People will be more willing to continue to be generous with you, and your gifts will provide an asset that leads to the abundance of others.

- By regularly sorting through household items that you no longer use, you clear space for yourself and provide resources to others. Place parameters around these items: Have you used them within a year? Do you have more than one? You can come up with your own standards. The bottom line is that if you don't need an item, your keeping it is stealing it from someone else in need. Donate it and know that you have helped someone else.

Again, the concept is that the more people have, the more they are likely to give. One scholarly study published by the Rotman School of Management found a correlation between feelings of deprivation and theft. It did not matter the material wealth of the individual; if that individual felt deprived in any way, he or she was more likely to steal and act immorally. The study concluded that feelings of lack or resentment led people to feel justified in taking.

Practicing yoga, especially focusing on *asteya*, eliminates these thoughts and feelings.

Joy and Emotional Resources as Energy

Money and other material goods are not the only sources of wealth. An individual who feels content and lives in the present moment is naturally inclined to practice *asteya*. In the same way that the transfer of physical property and currency flow (or are stuck due to a deficit mindset), so do emotions. It is easy to hold onto emotions that keep us stuck in a behavior pattern. When we act out of anything but the pure intentions of yoga, we rob ourselves and others of living this life with a clear heart-mind.

Citta-prasadana is the process of clarifying the heart-mind. It is a gradual practice of living in consciousness and the unification of the heart and mind to act as one clear, loving, and content being. We do this through many yoga practices, and *asteya* is a small conscious act that leads the way.

When we live in an unconscious manner, we say, do, and behave in ways that muddy the waters, stealing love, joy, and contentment. Here are ways in which we steal these precious resources:

- Clinging to the past or present deprives us and others of attention to the present moment.

- Focusing too heavily upon your own needs may distract you and put others in harmful situations.

- Holding onto judgements and prejudices robs others of their dignity. It also prevents you and others from sharing unique gifts and talents.

- Not speaking up when someone uses demeaning language toward others or participating in behaviors that disenfranchise others limits opportunities for the disempowered.

- Joining in on gossip or rejection of a person robs from their reputation and steals from relationships. People may not feel they can be their authentic self and that they are worthless.

- Interrupting conversations steals someone's ability to share what is on their mind and heart. It not only steals their time and platform, but it tells them they are not important enough to listen to.

The above list can become exhaustive as we participate in these activities willingly and without much thought. Even when we join in on common negative discussions about our spouses, family, in-laws, or even our own bodies, we are taking away from the divine aspects inherent in these beings.

Instead of participating in mindless chatter or belittling thoughts toward yourself and others, rewire your thoughts, words, and behavior patterns to reflect generous intentions:

- Change the topic of conversation from demoralizing to uplifting language. What does your spouse do right? How does a parent make the world better?

- Replace negative thoughts about your body and abilities. Focus on your attributes and how unique you are. Make goals and work toward them, knowing that you can reach them.

- When you hear racist, sexist, or any degrading dialogue that robs people of their human dignity, speak up. Stop these cycles of theft and don't participate.

- When you find yourself worrying about an event in the future or fretting over a decision you made in the past, gently bring your attention to the present. Use breath as your anchor. Feel your body. Listen to present conversations. Give your time and attention to the people and circumstances around you.

- Practice mindful listening. Listen to a conversation with the intent on listening, not on responding. Make eye contact and act in a way that says, "What you have to say is important to me."

Protecting the human dignity of others and their emotional resources will lead to supportive relationships, rooted in trust and inspiration. This action ensures people feel safe and secure in walking their life path and sharing their gifts with others. Opportunity and generosity will come to you in many ways, both in service and support.

How Can *Asteya* Lead to an Accumulation of Wealth?

Moral integrity and protecting others' possessions, time, and dignity does more than make you feel good. Consistently ethical behavior that works to protect others will lead to many opportunities to accumulate abundance and comfort.

When you desire what others have, you can waste your time and money trying to compare. Instead, when you defend what others have and find joy in their fortune, you can find yourself in situations that lead to wealth. For example, if you are in a management position, and you are put in charge of others' possessions, they must trust you. If they don't, you lose your job. If they do, then you will continue to earn a salary and save for your own possessions.

When you choose to judge others and treat them in a demeaning way, you close yourself off to their gifts. Instead, if you honor people for who they are, you get to know and understand them. They may open up to you and provide you with gifts you never imagined. For example, if a person who provides a valuable service (cleaning, baking, painting houses, fixing cars, etc.) feels safe and valued in your presence, you may be able to barter for their skills. They may have an answer for you that solves a problem you've been dealing with. Either way, they most likely will save you money and time (and you may earn a friend).

When you live with a scarcity mindset, feeling deprived and desperate, then you may turn to stealing to fulfill your needs. Clinging to other people's possessions will not bring you abundance; it will bring you heartache and emptiness. Instead, if you practice gratitude, you can turn your focus toward creating more abundance for yourself and others. When you are grateful for your job, you are willing to put in the work necessary to reach your goals, which will lead to a consistent salary. When you are grateful for material goods, you will take care of them, and they will serve their purpose. When you are grateful for other people, you nurture an environment in which they feel safe to share their time, talents, and possessions.

Asteya asks us to protect people, in their wealth and joy. But most importantly, it asks us to protect the unique path each of us walk while inhabiting this planet, making it work for the benefit of us all.

4

Aparigrahā: How the Practice of Non-Hoarding Can Benefit Your Wallet and Illuminate Your Path

"When non-greed is confirmed, a thorough illumination of the how and why of one's birth comes."
-The Yoga Sūtra of Patāñjali, 2.39

Attachment is the root of all suffering. The world's greatest spiritual leaders and innovative thinkers agree that to cling to anything is a detriment to one's quality of life. When we fear losing something, when we divert all our resources toward accumulation, or when we obsess over any temporary earthly possession, we commit a tremendous disservice to our life's purpose: To Be.

Any number of material possessions, including life itself, can be the epicenter of focus, detracting from serious self-development:

- Physical appearance of the body

- Title and social status

- Fixation on power, prestige, and reputation

- Bank account balance

- House size and vehicle model

- Collection of valuables, memorabilia, and heirlooms

- Clothing, shoes, and apparel accumulation

Humans have the potential to hoard literally any possession, idea, and source of abundance. This hoarding can lead to a host of issues, to include

- Diminished resources for those in need

- Unhealthy attachment to material possessions and the ego (identity)

- Crippling anxiety over the loss of life or reputation

- Alienating friends, family, and coworkers by dominating conversations and ignoring the ideas of others

- Feeling obligated to reciprocate, instead of giving and receiving freely

- Maintaining rigid ideas and opinions, even to the detriment of one's health and safety

- Living a life out of alignment with one's purpose and gifts

These consequences bring us misery in the form of isolation, despair, and meaninglessness. When we act from the ego, we distort consciousness. Living a life according to the *sūtras* and practicing *aparigrahā* (non-hoarding) will provide a clear lens through which to inform our actions.

What is *Aparigrahā* and How Does It Lead to Wealth?

In Sanskrit, *aparigrahā* translates to "non-hoarding". Ironically, letting go is the key to abundance. Think about a water faucet. If you keep it turned off, tightly, it will not produce water. You may think you are saving water this way, or you may be trying to lower your utility bill, but by preventing the flow of water, you are depriving yourself of essential hydration. It isn't wise to hoard water. People need it to survive. We should maintain water sources, nourish our bodies, and share our supplies with others.

Everything works this way: money, clothing, shelter, advice, love, and even time. Nothing can be gathered, stored, and securely locked away. When we act in this way, we keep that which we withhold from serving its purpose. Preventing the flow of generosity, benefit, and divine design is not only unwise, it is what keeps us enslaved to the very possessions we hold so dear. By holding tightly to anything, we diminish its worth and prevent blessings from flowing our way.

Clinging to Life

The most common attachment we have is to our body, our life. This clinging is understandable, since it is the vehicle of existence. If the body is unwell, it is difficult to manage daily responsibilities and interactions. If the body is dead, well, then that is the end of the journey. It is scary to be sick or to face death. But clinging to life—the ego—provides us with a false sense of identity. We are not the body! We are Awareness, itself.

The ego is the human way of creating an identity. *I am a teacher. I am a writer. I am a person.* All of these labels describe what *I* do or how *I* think of *myself*. But when we label and identify with such roles, we create boundaries

217

between ourselves and others. We are not separate, and we are not composed of these superficial circumstances. Even the words "I" and "mine" can be dangerous to realizing that which liberates. When we eliminate the labels and the ego's insatiable need to be central to all decision making, then we take a step toward freedom.

What happens when we allow the ego to make decisions? We fall prey to outcomes. We worry so much about the destination that we lose sight of the journey. We worry so much about losing life that we forget to live. We worry so much about the appearance of the body that we neglect our soul.

How to Practice Non-Attachment to the Body

The body is a vehicle. It houses the Awareness that is us: the mind, emotions, and consciousness. It converts food into fuel. It moves us. It embraces our loved ones. It gives us an experience, here on Earth. We worry a lot about our bodies. We worry about past choices that have led to regret. We worry about the future and its potential consequences. But there are a few practices we can maintain that help the body remain present, really the only moment that exists.

Non-attachment through movement. Whether walking, running, swimming, or *āsana*, exercise is an excellent way to

218

maintain presence. Feel the body move. Focus on the breath. Exercising in nature may add tremendous benefit to your routine. If you're practicing yoga, remain barefooted and in the process. The most important part of the workout is to eliminate self-criticism or competitiveness with others. Let go of the outcome and enjoy the ride.

Non-attachment through diet. Sometimes, eating becomes a means to comfort rather than for sustenance. It is easy to over-indulge if we are feeling emotionally vulnerable. Sometimes, people behave in the opposite way, eating too little, because their attachment to the idea of a perfect body prevents them from enjoying a balanced diet. Further, hoarding food can lead to food waste. About 1.3 billion tons of food is wasted each year, globally, which amounts to a third of all food produced. Unless it is an extreme situation, buy only what you need and make a plan to purchase food that supports a healthy diet (not one that feeds an alternative need).

Non-attachment through acceptance. The ego naturally feels as if it never has enough. It is competitive and obsessed with reputation. It is the reason we buy the clothing, cars, and homes we do. Often, we do not buy out of a sense of practicality and necessity, but rather, we make purchases that will enhance our image. We overwork our bodies—stress our emotional, mental, and physical systems—for power and prestige. We worry about titles. When we practice *aparigrahā*, we practice contentment (*saṁtoṣa*, which is another *niyama*). Accepting what is opens us up to realizing blessings, without the distraction of worry.

Clinging to Possessions

One of the easiest resources to hold onto is money. Saving money is important. It is a good idea to have a source of money for emergencies, for when you can no longer work (sick or retired), or to purchase a necessity. But when we over-save, clinging to money, we deprive ourselves in many ways. At this point, we go from prudent saving to hoarding.

In the same way, we can hold onto a job that doesn't serve our purpose, because we are afraid to lose money or other benefits. We may collect items we do not need or refuse to let go of material possessions due to an emotional attachment, which turns into hoarding.

Greed can also turn into over-consumption and unfair market practices. When people act out of greed, they prevent the flow of abundance to those in need. We see this with oil accumulation and production, the high cost of medication, and commercials aimed at creating a constant desire for more of the latest gadgets.

How to Practice Non-Attachment to Possessions

While many of us don't have control over the actions of others, we can control our own behaviors regarding greed and attachment.

Non-attachment through use of money. Money, like all sources of energy, is meant to flow. This action does not mean that you overspend or use money unwisely; what it does mean is that you should use it to better yourself and others, and not hoard it. What does maintaining an open flow of money look like?

- Invest in yourself through purchasing what inspires you: books, art supplies, music, a gym membership, a new tool, a trip to a desired destination, and more. It is not a blank check to buy whatever you want; it is an open invitation to support your body, mind, and spirit.

- Support others through monetary gifts. Give a small monthly donation to a charity of your choice. Purchase a few extra boxes of non-perishable food for groceries to donate to the local food bank. Also, accept gifts freely without feeling obligated to the giver. This acceptance is an important aspect of *aparigrahā*.

- Keep saving but save for the right reasons. It is still important to put money aside for emergencies, repairs, larger purchases, retirement, higher education, etc. Don't simply hold onto money, put money away intentionally.

Non-attachment through finding purpose. It is easy to work at a job you hate. Maybe you feel as if you are in the wrong profession, entirely. It's difficult to give up years of experience and education to try something more rewarding. In the same light, you may be working for the paycheck or health insurance, but at the risk of your mental, physical, and emotional health. Without putting yourself and others in jeopardy, realize that holding tight to a job that does not highlight your purpose or gifts can be damaging. An unhealthy attachment to daily work that hurts you, rather than helps, can prevent you from actualizing your true potential. And your potential is a gift to the world.

Non-attachment through sharing resources. Many people hoard resources, and they may not be aware of it. Shopping in bulk may be necessary for your family or make sense financially, but over-buying can diminish your monetary resources, perpetuate feelings that you never have enough, and keep valuable resources away from those who need it most.

Additionally, you may hold onto shoes, clothes, and other possessions that you haven't used in years, simply because you are afraid to let go. Continually not using an item means you don't need it, and it is time to clear your clutter so these items can be put to better use.

- Turn all the hangers around in your closet. When you wear an item, turn it again, and keep it that way for the remainder of the year. If a hanger is left unturned at the end of a year, donate it. You can do the same thing with shoes, jewelry, or other items.

- Only purchase what you need. If you prefer to shop in bulk for cost savings or to eliminate trips to the store, this action can be a smart idea. Do not, however, buy more than is practical. These extra items take up space, limit resources from others, and take money out of your paycheck. Holding onto unused items also requires maintenance, which further wastes your time and money.

- As discussed earlier, food waste is an enormous problem. If you have food that may expire (but hasn't already) or if you identify a food item you know you won't need, donate it. If you garden, give a portion of your produce to a food bank that accepts fresh produce (or can your goods). Contact and help a local bakery distribute older baked goods to homebound individuals.

Clinging to Ideas

Anxiety disorders, which include generalized anxiety disorder (GAD) obsessive-compulsive disorder (OCD), post-traumatic stress disorder (PTSD), and social anxiety disorder (SAD), are the most common mental afflictions affecting adults in the United States. Nearly 40 million adults in the U.S. struggle with life-altering behaviors due to anxiety. Anxiety-related symptoms include overthinking, clinging to rigid beliefs, and living in a state of fear or panic. A person doesn't even have to be diagnosed with any anxiety disorder to suffer from mental overload and stress.

Religion, politics, and personality can also create fixed and inflexible belief systems. Humans naturally create boundaries among each other, and ideological fences are at the root of most conflicts. Clinging to rigid ideas and beliefs can limit personal growth, hurt and prevent healing relationships, and keep people from actualizing important "truths". Of course, we do not know what is true, except that open hearts and minds lead to liberation from untruths.

Obsession is yet another form of overthinking. Humans obsess over money, time, and relationships. When we constantly think of one person, place, thing, or idea, we rob ourselves of seeing anything else of worth in our lives. Clinging to time—to the past or future—also robs us of the present moment. When we form unhealthy attachments to ruminating about the past or worrying about the future, valuable Presence eludes us.

Non-attachment through listening. One way that we hoard is through ignoring others' ideas and interrupting during conversations. As mentioned in an earlier chapter, interrupting is also a form of theft (the remedy is *asteya*). Often, leaders neglect sharing power, because they are afraid it will make them look weak. Non-attachment to power and control will open any process up to innovation and solutions. Listening to people is a way to add to your life, and it may increase the potential to save and earn money.

Non-attachment through learning. *Svādhyāya* is also one of the *niyamas* and is the practice of improvement through independent study. Reading about different cultures, particularly ancient texts, is an excellent way to open the flow of resources. Understanding other cultural practices, languages, and beliefs creates opportunity for experience and collaboration. Seeing things from another angle, whether through *svādhyāya* or *āsana*, will take you to places unavailable before.

Non-attachment through Presence. Hoarding ideas through overthinking can prevent the flow of innovation as well as create anxiety, depression, and other body-mind afflictions. When we ruminate over past decisions, we neglect the important work that must be done today. When we worry too much about the future, we spend our time lost in thought rather than productive action. Mindfulness can lead to increased productivity, adaptability, and creativity. We can remain present through the following behaviors:

- Try not to multitask. Maintain focus (*dṛṣṭi*) and resources on one task, creating meaningful processes and outcomes.

- Practice mindfulness. Use the senses to be in the moment—pay attention to sights, smells, skin sensations, tastes, and sounds—even during mundane chores.

- Incorporate yogic and Ayurvedic practices into your day. Breathwork (*prāṇāyāma*), daily hygiene routines (*dinacharyā*), *sattvic* diet, and exercise (*āsana*) can help manage stress and keep you healthy, which keeps you working.

Attachments block the flow of energy. Holding too tightly to life, possessions, and ideas inhibits creativity, problem solving, and sharing resources, which supports others. When we share of ourselves—our time, talents, and material goods—we benefit the world. Other people will want to share with us. Supporting someone else may help improve their circumstances, which will ultimately benefit you. When we make a choice to let go of attachments, we stop hoarding abundance. If we aren't buying more than we need, we save money and realize opportunity. To practice *aparigrahā* is to tap into and open the flow of life's blessings.

5

Sādhana: How Consistent Practice Creates a Strong Foundation for an Abundant

"They help us minimize obstacles and obtain Samādhi."
-The Yoga Sūtra of Patāñjali, 2.2

Most people have heard about the parable of the house built on the rock. To remain stable and to flourish, it is necessary to take great strides toward building a strong foundation. Adversely, it is the fool who builds upon weak and loose foundation (the sand), hastily constructing without persistent planning. Deliberate and consistent practice leads to the rewards of building upon the rock, living a life that is pure and void of the obstacles that prevent joy, peace, and stability.

A consistent yoga practice is such a dedicated practice. When one lives the eight-limbed path of *Aṣṭāṅga Yoga*, one builds a steady, undisturbed, and untarnished foundation: physically, mentally, emotionally, and spiritually. It is not that one achieves perfection—that is impossible. However, it is possible to cultivate abundance in strength of the heart-mind-body with dedication and discipline to the tenets of this path.

Aṣṭāṅga Yoga is not the only path and type of yoga, however. Many variations and schools of yoga exist. Historically, the *Yoga Sūtras* are the primary text of *Rāja Yoga*, which translates to 'the science of the mind". These threads were written over a period from 5,000 BCE to 300 CE. It is unclear if the author is a person named Patāñjali or if several people contributed to this text; however, this writing acts to organize the practices already in existence. As the modern world evolved, so did the experience of yoga, which can be practiced in the following ways:

- *Hatha Yoga* = yoga of postures

- *Rāja Yoga* = yoga of self-control

- *Kuṇḍalinī Yoga* = yoga of energy

- *Karma Yoga* = yoga of mind

- *Jñāna Yoga* = yoga of Self-inquiry

- *Bhakti Yoga* = yoga of devotion

Regardless of one's intention, interest, or ability, a consistent personal practice (*sādhana*) will strengthen and support the foundation from which life takes root. Poor health, decision making, emotional regulation, and other aspects can interfere with wellness. If one builds upon a steady rock, these obstacles disappear, leading the practitioner down the path toward health, wealth, and relationship. It is through maintaining these various aspects of our lives that we realize true abundance.

What is *Sādhana* and How Does It Lead to Abundance?

In Sanskrit, *sādhana* translates to "spiritual practice". The reason why yoga, in its many forms, is considered a spiritual practice is because its ultimate transformation leads to union with all of consciousness (including divine consciousness). *Sādhana* is the means of accomplishing this union. One can get there through the discipline of practicing yoga, as described in any one of its contemporary schools. However, to keep in alignment with the basics of this book, one's life can be vastly supported through practicing the *yamas, niyamas, āsana, prāṇāyāma, pratyāhāra, dhāraṇā, dhyāna,* and *Samādhi*.

Practice leads to steadiness, experience, and skill. These qualities lead to prosperity. In the beginning, though, practice is not always easy. As we introduce the body, mind, and spirit to rigor, they often rebel. The body is full of toxins from poor diet and exercise habits. The mind is full of toxic thoughts and obsessions from inner and outer influences. The spirit is full of toxins from the suffering and separation from our Source, the divine consciousness that resides in us all. These toxins or obstructions (*kleśas*) prevent us from obtaining peace, stability, and joy. Through *sādhana*, one may eliminate the obstructions to a better life.

How *Sādhana* Supports Abundance through Physical Health

"Āsana is a steady, comfortable posture."
-The Yoga Sūtra of Patāñjali, 2.46

The body is an imperfect vehicle. Maybe it is riddled with dis-ease and ailments from chronic afflictions. These afflictions can be purely physical (hereditary or harmful habits) or they can stem from the effects of harbored and stagnant mental and emotional afflictions. Everything affects the body. Even in a relatively healthy person, the body is not symptom free. Aging and strain can cause aches and pains. Poor diet and exercise can cause digestive problems, or worse, chronic and life-threatening illnesses, such as cancer or diabetes.

Whatever may afflict the body, these issues can impede performance, which can ultimately lead to diminished resources:

- Dis-ease and illness can prevent people from working, thus receiving necessary wages.

- Chronic or acute illness may require clinic or hospital visits, which lead to considerable medical bills, including the cost of prescription drugs.

- Poor health can lead to higher health insurance premiums and other related costs.

A lifetime of ill health can lead to an overall lack of abundance. When people are unable to work or cannot work at the capacity of their healthier counterparts, they are unable to save and use their money toward wealth generation. Being financially unstable can lead one to purchase cheaper, yet inadequate food supplies. It may lead to more distress, which can lead to a host of other physical issues, possibly even substance abuse or mental/emotional afflictions. Neglecting the body is the first step toward neglecting the foundation.

Adversely, being devoted to the health of the body will improve the longevity and quality of life, as well as increase financial circumstances. In many traditions, the body is considered a temple for the spirit. It is the vehicle from which our thoughts and emotions are housed. The quality of your mental and emotional faculties are in alignment with the health of the body. Further, when the body dies, life ends for that aspect of consciousness. For these reasons, maintaining, and even beautifying, the body can be a spiritual practice.

Sādhana in Action

It is one thing to read about yoga, and even practice its tenets. But it is another to put your personal spiritual practice into action. This action is often referred to as *kriyā*, which translates to "action or practice". It is not enough to simply eat healthy or exercise; if one wants to build a solid foundation from within to change the world without, then one must approach this holy temple with actionable and spiritual intention.

- Cultivate a spiritual practice that is right for you. Consistency is the key to building a strong foundation.

  - Start the day with a hygiene routine (mentioned in earlier chapters), gentle *āsana*, and a calming meditation.

○ Eat a diet that is responsibly sourced and one that supports physical wellbeing.

○ Be mindful about any substance that goes into your body.

○ Spend time outdoors, especially in nature. Our bodies are like plants; we need sun, water, fresh air, and earth.

○ Get adequate amounts of water and sleep.

○ Balance rest with movement, work with pleasure, discipline with release.

○ Infuse every action with love, gratitude, and unity (*Samādhi*).

When every action becomes holy, you build your temple on a rock. A strong foundation will lead to fewer illnesses and dis-ease, which will lead to fewer medical expenses. A healthy body is also a body that can act, whether it be working, recreating, or advocating for others. But remember, it is okay to rest and take time off from your rituals, a sort of abstinence. The body needs recharging, and it is important to listen to its needs without guilt or shame.

This is the practice of *ahiṁsā* in action: Non-injury toward oneself.

How *Sādhana* Supports Abundance through Mental Health

"The restraint of the modifications of the mind-stuff is Yoga."
-The Yoga Sūtra of Patāñjali, 1.2

Mental health is not a secondary concern, nor is it separate from the body's health. How the mind operates affects the health of the body, and the health of the body affects the operation of the mind. As noted earlier, the *Yoga Sūtras* are the systemization of the practices of *Rāja Yoga*. As explained in the introduction of "The Yoga Sūtras of Patāñjali", this "mental science" (p. xi) describes a process of observation, discernment, and discipline of the mind. The practitioner turns within to study one's own consciousness, working to control its impulses and impurities. The outcome creates a clear lens from which to view the inner and outer worlds, and the desired result should lead to a calm and content demeanor.

Unfortunately, life is not that simple, and the mind, in its unbridled state, is unsteady. "Your values may change within a fraction of a second," says Śrī Svāmī Saccidānanda as he expands upon *Sūtra* 1.2 (p. 5). The quality of everything is a construct of the mind: time, relationships, and even your own personality. For this reason, it is essential to detach from these projections and mental modifications.

The brain is a magnificent organ. Its job is to make sense of sensory input and make sense of its surroundings. But its blessing can also be its curse in that it literally has a mind of its own. As is a common description of *citta*, this monkey mind screams for your attention. It is always seeking, it is always contemplating, it obsesses and diverts your attention to any shiny object that gets its attention. For this reason, people suffer. They are in bondage to the whims of the mind.

- Clinging to the past can make a person regretful and depressed.

- Worrying about the future can make a person fearful and anxious.

- Obsessive thoughts can override necessary and important decision making.

- Distraction can diminish productivity.

- Attachment to outside influences can create emotions, such as rage, jealousy, or judgment that obstruct productivity and prosperity.

- Building a life (purchases, behaviors, etc.) based on external perceptions can thwart the ability to provide based on needs and destroy contentment.

Mental liberation starts with oneself. It is through changing that one can find contentment, even joy, in everyday life. *Sādhana* is a means of accomplishing this liberation. Dedication to the inward journey, to creating a clear heart-mind, is the ultimate homage to the divine consciousness. It is through controlling the individual consciousness that one affects the collect, and it is through this action that one demonstrates devotion to the divine consciousness.

Sādhana in Action

Control of the mind is the most effective path toward making decisions that build a healthy and strong foundation. When one is liberated from addictions, desires, and attachment to the physical world, the body can thrive. When one lives in acceptance and eliminates judgments based on duality (good vs. bad), then one can remain calm throughout any circumstances. It is through this vantage point that one makes prudent decisions that lead to abundance on every level.

- A devout spiritual practice that nourishes the mental faculties will lead to prosperity:

    o Begin each day with a prayer or reverence for all which you are grateful to have. Gratitude can rewire the brain to see the positive aspects of any situation.

    o Commit to a regular meditation practice. Physically, meditation can help the body regulate hormone release, as well as respiratory and circulatory function. Mentally, meditation helps to eliminate symptoms of anxiety and depression, and it boosts memory and concentration. Meditation is also a spiritual act, as it is the means *Samādhi* through *dhāraṇā* and *dhyāna*.

    o Check your daily habits: Diet, exercise, and substance use can all affect cognition, concentration, and mood. Regular deep breathing and concentrated breathing (*prāṇāyāma*) can help calm the mind of its incessant chatter (*citta*).

○ Regularly practice mindfulness. Presence is the time to live. Everything else is a mental construct. Intentional focus is a means to control sensory judgments. Through *pratyāhāra*, we can lean more on our intuition and less on external input.

The mind is the master. Where we focus our attention is how we communicate with everything around us. If we focus on negative outcomes, negative outcomes we will attract. Fear makes us hold tightly to that which we have and prevents us from taking important steps toward prosperity. Directing our focus on what we hate about ourselves and others makes us see those traits as reality. However, if we focus on the positive, the God-in-everything, we not only uplift the mood, but we transform the mind into a magnet of abundance. How? Trust, forgiveness, and non-attachment lead to courage, acceptance, and contentment. Taking control of the mind, so the mind does not control you, is a spiritual imperative to move you toward rewarding decision making.

How *Sādhana* Supports Abundance through Spiritual Health

"Those who merely leave their physical bodies and attain the state of celestial deities, or those who get merged in Nature, have rebirth."
-The Yoga Sūtra of Patañjali, 1.19

Cultivating a devout spiritual practice is rewarding in many ways. As Śrī Svāmī Saccidānanda repeatedly emphasizes, one does not need to meditate for hours a day to achieve spiritual liberation. Each action rooted in yoga can become a personal *sādhana*. Some people achieve great levels of control over their lives. Some achieve deep and profound levels of *Samādhi*. Yet, perfection is impossible, because we are human. The journey, the process, and the practice are the point. Rebirth occurs when we evolve, whether that is in one action, one lifetime, or a continuous cycle of death and rebirth. A strong spiritual foundation leads to great gains:

- Numerous empirical studies suggest that people who regularly participate in spiritual practices suffer less from anxiety, depression, and overall dis-ease.

- Spiritual fitness is steeped in the tenets of kindness, compassion, and forgiveness, all of which lead to positive inner peace and outer interactions.

- Connecting with our spiritual centers provides meaning to our existence, which helps us identify and live with purpose.

Sādhana in Action

Establishing a personal spiritual practice may be easy or difficult depending on one's upbringing and life experience. Religion can either be a positive or negative experience, but spiritual connection—authentic inner love and commitment—provides us with tools to live in peace. When we shed the desires of this physical world, yet treat all with holy reverence, we see the benefit of every manifestation. A goodness that informs our everyday actions.

- Spiritual health is found inside each of us, and the path is a personal journey:

    ○ Create a sacred space (or several) to which you can demonstrate your devotion. Decorate with items that are symbolic and sacred, such as candles, pieces of nature, and reminders of one's deity.

241

○ Use prayer as a method of communication with what you are devoted to. Prayer is a mindful way to contemplate, request, and display gratitude.

○ Chanting, singing, dancing, and other movements are excellent ways to feel into your own spirituality. These forms of energy are sacred and uplifting.

○ Spend time in Nature. Infuse your life with the elements of the Universe: water, earth, ether, fire, and air. Source energy is in all, and reverence to these life-sustaining resources can be great reminders of all we have.

A personal *sādhana* is a gift. It is the way to a strong foundation, inside and out. It is a gentle reminder that all is sacred and of one consciousness. It is a grounding yet uplifting means to accomplish greatness. The steadiness of one's "house" is a solace to the world. Let your light shine from every window.

Namaste

Supplemental
Material

What is *Āyurveda* and How Does It Work?

Āyurveda has become a popular buzzword among health-conscious communities—a mysterious and trendy holistic healing hype. But *Āyurveda* is not new nor trendy: It is a lifestyle choice that was developed thousands of years ago. So, what is *Āyurveda*, and how does it work to promote health and healing? With a few key foundational concepts, anyone can obtain and use the wisdom that is *Āyurveda*.

What is *Āyurveda*?

Āyurveda is a sister science of yoga. Both yoga and *Āyurveda* were developed in India thousands of years ago and are rooted in Vedic texts. While *veda* means 'knowledge", *ayur* means 'life". Therefore, *Āyurveda* literally translates from Sanskrit as 'life knowledge". Today, *Āyurveda* has been modernized, not only in India, but also in the United States, where it has become a part of yogic practice.

An Ayurvedic lifestyle consists of principles and practices that will enhance health, with a focus on preventing and healing dis-ease. It's important to recognize the term dis-ease not as pathological illness (disease) but rather that of a lack of ease. By forging a life knowledge of natural remedies—foods, herbs, rituals, etc.—alongside an

244

understanding of natural rhythms, anyone can live an Ayurvedic lifestyle.

How Does *Āyurveda* Work?

To begin understanding how *Āyurveda* works, it is important to learn about *Āyurvedic doshas*. In the West, the term *dosha* has become a popular way to describe an individual's energy that governs the body. However, a more appropriate term to use is *Prakṛiti*, which is Sanskrit for "nature". Prakṛiti is the natural composition of energy, the matter that makes up anything. To elaborate, each person has a natural constitution that affects health. *Dosha* comes from the Sanskrit term *doṣa*, which translates to "that which spoils". For simplicity, and because much information available to the West uses this term, we will use *dosha* to explain the constitutions.

What are *Āyurveda Doshas*?

When we think about our *doshas*, we must think about what energy is most prevalent in our bodies. The key objective in *Āyurveda* is to balance those energies. The three *Āyurveda* doshas are

- *Kapha*

- *Pitta*

- *Vata*

Everyone's' life-energy consists of all three *doshas*, but everyone will be made up of different proportions of them. Some people can be mostly one, mostly two (with the third lacking), or tridoshic—an equal balance of all three.

The most important step in understanding and using *Āyurveda* in your life is to identify and understand your *dosha*(s). The best method to determine this information is with an *Āyurveda* lifestyle consultation. Many consultants exist, especially in yogic and holistic health communities. However, to start, it is possible to begin learning about your dosha by taking an online quiz, like one through Banyan Botanical, which is a reputable source.

Doshas are sourced from the five states of matter: earth, water, air, fire, and ether (space). *Kapha* is a combination of earth and water; *pitta* is a combination of fire and water; and *vata* is a combination of air and ether. Each *dosha* has its presence in your body and governs different aspects of your physical, mental, and emotional composition, as well as overall health. Below are characteristics, attributes, and qualities of the *doshas*:

Kapha

- This combination of water and earth has to do with the body's overall structure. Water and earth bind, and so in the body, *kapha* is the energy that binds cells, bones, muscle, and fat. Its purpose is to protect the body. Qualities include oily, solid, heavy, slow, grounded, and cool.

- Emotionally and mentally, individuals with a primary *kapha* constitution are loving, calm, and considerate. If balanced, they are loyal, consistent, and fun-loving. Excess *kapha* can lead to feelings of insecurity, attachment, and depression.

- Physically, individuals with a primary *kapha* constitution are strong and exhibit qualities consistent with moisture: lubricated eyes, skin, and thick, healthy hair. If balanced, they have sound digestion and sleep patterns. Excess *kapha* can lead to issues with the lungs and weight.

Pitta

- This combination of fire and water has to do with the body's digestion and production of energy (including metabolism). Fire and water burn and evaporate, and so in the body, pitta is the energy that transforms. Qualities include penetrating, intense, light, fast, pungent, and hot.

- Emotionally and mentally, individuals with a primary *pitta* constitution are passionate, and have a sharp intellect and focus. If balanced, they are great decision-makers, orators, and teachers. Excess *pitta* can lead to a hot temper and argumentative nature.

- Physically, individuals with a primary *pitta* constitution have a medium body type and exhibit qualities consistent with heat: baldness or reddish hair, exuberance, strong sex drive, warm body temperature, and a strong appetite. If balanced, they will have excellent digestion and polished skin. Excess *pitta* can lead to inflammation, indigestion, ulcers, and skin rashes.

Vata

- This combination of air and ether has to do with vital body functions and the flow of the nervous system. Air and ether move energy, and so in the body, *vata* is the energy that moves breath, blood, and waste. Qualities include dry, rough, quick, irregular, changeable, and cold.

- Emotionally and mentally, individuals with a primary *vata* constitution are curious, creative, and dynamic. If balanced, they are inventive, flexible, and apt to take initiative. Excess *vata* can lead to insomnia, anxiety, and inability to cope with stress.

- Physically, individuals with a primary *vata* constitution have a light and agile body, and exhibit qualities consistent with air: energetic, excitable, and dry/cool hair and skin. They are light sleepers. Excess *vata* can lead to fatigue, weakness, hypertension, weight loss, and digestive sensitivities.

How Do I Balance My *Dosha*?

The primary goal of Ayurvedic medicine is to balance the presence of your energy and not accumulate an excess of one specific energy. It is worth noting that the energy of each season of the year and time of day is consistent with the three *doshas*. So, while you can act in accordance with recommendations for your particular constitution, you will also need to take the season and time of day into consideration for optimal wellness and healing (see below for information about seasonal and daily routines).

How does *Āyurveda* heal? According to this life knowledge, like energy increases like energy and opposites cure. For example, if you are an individual with a primary *pitta* constitution, and you are experiencing hot flashes, indigestion, and inflammation (skin, joints, veins, etc.), then you will want to avoid spicy and pungent foods, like tomatoes and peppers. Or you will want to avoid hot exercises, like *Aṣṭāṅga Yoga* (*āsana*) or high-intensity interval training (HIIT). Instead, you will most likely benefit from oily and cool foods, using coconut oil and aloe juice to chill your digestive fire. Additionally, you would want to engage in meditation and *Yin Yoga* to keep you cool. Below is a more specific *Āyurveda* beginners guide for each *dosha*.

How Do I Balance My *Kapha Dosha*?

As with mud (water and earth), excess *kapha* can slow energy. It is essential that individuals with excess *kapha* work to negate its effect to balance their constitution, with the primary goal to provide and move energy:

- Stimulate your body with regular exercise.

- Seek warm and dry environments.

- Engage in activities that stimulate your mind as well as your body.

- Adhere to a diet and exercise routine that limits excess *kapha*.

- Avoid clutter and congestion in your life.

- Use vibrant music, and warm colors and aromas for stimulation (see Additional Suggestions section below).

- Manage your sleep schedule by waking before 6 a.m. each day and avoiding naps.

- Make sure to use a neti pot and dry brushing in your daily routine.

Recommended Exercises for *Kapha*

Pick an exercise routine that is warming and stimulating:

- *Aṣṭāṅga Yoga* and hot yoga practices are great methods to keep *kapha* moving. *

- Breathing exercises, such as *Kapalabhati* (skull-shining breath), that add stimulation and heat to your daily routine.

Recommended Diet for *Kapha*

Choose foods that are light, warming, and have limited moisture. A good *kapha* diet should keep these goals in mind:

- Eat plenty of fruits and vegetables.

- Use warm spices (limiting salt).

- Avoid dairy, nuts, and seeds.

- Limit red meats and oily foods; try cooking with extra virgin olive oil, sunflower oil, or ghee.

How Do I Balance My *Pitta Dosha*?

As with evaporation (fire and water), excess *pitta* simultaneously consumes and feeds energy (think water dropped on a hot pan). It is essential that individuals with excess *pitta* work to negate the effects of their heat, working toward cooling and stabilizing their energy:

- Balance priorities and rest. Do not burn yourself out.

- Keep a consistent eating schedule. Both skipping meals and over-indulging will create excess digestive heat.

- Adhere to diet and exercise that limit accumulation of excess *pitta*.

- Don yourself with cool colors, enjoy cooling and sweet aromas, and listen to calming music.

- Take regular walks in nature, specifically spending time near bodies of water. Moon bathe.

- Incorporate laughter and joy into your day.

- Use self-massage with cooling oils (coconut or olive) as a part of your daily routine.

Recommended Exercises for *Pitta*

Avoid exercise routines that will add excess heat to your body. While it is important to enjoy cardio workouts for health, keep your time in these activities to the bare minimum.

- Swimming increases cardio, enhances muscle strength, and beats the heat.

- Perform *Chandra Namaskara* (Moon Salutations) that cool.

- Yoga twists and bends release tension and lymph, which create heat.

- Open the heart (think compassion and patience) with chest openers, such as *Uṣṭrāsana* (Camel Pose).

- Meditate regularly and engage in *Sitali Prāṇāyāma* (cooling breath) to prevent and reduce heat.

Recommended Diet for *Pitta*

Choose foods that are pacifying to *pitta,* which are cooling, sweet, and bitter (yes, both!).

- Avoid sour, salty, and pungent foods, and this includes dairy. Fermented foods may add more digestive fire than desired.

- Limit intake of hot vegetables, like garlic, peppers, and onion.

- Use honey and molasses as a natural sweetener, and indulge in sweet fruits, such as mangoes, melons, pineapples.

- Avoid corn byproducts or brown rice, and increase intake of barley and oats.

- Lubricate your system by cooking with oils and ghee. Use cooling oils, like sunflower, coconut, or olive. Avoid warming oils like corn, sesame, and almond.

How Do I Balance My *Vata Dosha*?

As with wind (air and ether), excess *vata* can over stimulate energy movement. It is essential that individuals with excess *vata* work to negate the effects of their constant movement, which can lead to anxiety, insomnia, and unintended weight loss.

- Slow down. Meditate or sit quietly, especially when feelings of mental, emotional, and physical speed affect your life.

- Eat regular meals, in accordance with a vata pacifying diet.

255

- Go to bed before 10 p.m., and do not sleep past 6 a.m.

- Keep a consistent schedule or daily routine.

- Avoid chilly places and be prepared in cold weather with a head covering and sweater.

- Incorporate warming self-massages into your daily routine, with use of sesame or almond oil.

- Adhere to an exercise regimen that limits excess *vata*.

- Use warm colors, as well as sweet and heavy aromas to soothe. Calming music is also beneficial.

- Be certain to eliminate body waste regularly. Add ginger tea to your diet.

Recommended Exercises for *Vata*

Adopt a light exercise routine with a focus on increasing flexibility and balance. Make certain not to push yourself too hard. People with a *vata* imbalance can easily fatigue and are prone to weight loss.

- Optimal activities for *vata* include golf, tennis, talking, Tai Chi, yoga, dance, and light hiking/biking.

- Grounding poses, such as *Tāḍāsana* (Mountain Pose) and inversions are great for keeping vata stable and balanced.

Recommended Diet for *Vata*

Sweet foods pacify *vata* but pay attention to intake. It is important for people with *vata* constitutions to eat larger quantities to keep up with their constant movement (but be mindful not to overeat).

- Incorporate healthy fats and oils, like ghee and extra virgin olive oil, to aid digestion.

- Eat rice and wheat, and eat less barley, corn, or rye.

- Consume low-fat dairy. Warm milk is pacifying to *vata*.

- Increase intake of nuts, cooked vegetables, and heavier fruits (bananas, avocados, coconut, and dry fruits)

- Avoid beans, except for mung bean (an *Āyurvedic* staple) and tofu.

- Add warm spices to cooking, such as oregano, cardamom, basil, and thyme.

What is an *Āyurvedic* Diet?

In *Āyurveda*, food is medicine. Some foods aggravate and some pacify. It is important to choose an Ayurvedic diet that pacifies. You can choose tridoshic foods (foods that pacify all three *doshas*) or foods that negate or oppose the qualities of your specific *dosha* (i.e. *kapha* and *vata* should choose warming foods, while *pitta* should choose cooling). Here are some staples of an Ayurvedic diet:

Ghee is a mega food. Also known as clarified butter, it helps to fight inflammation, can improve digestion, and can enhance your immunity.

Sesame oil is tridoshic. Although *pitta* should use it sparingly because of its warmth, and *kapha* should use it sparingly because of its heaviness, sesame oil works to pacify all doshas.

Yellow mung dal is a split lentil that makes many basic and essential Āyurvedic dishes. Try a general moong dal recipe or kitchari.

Herbs are important in an Ayurvedic diet. You can use them in cooking as well as in teas. More information about specific *Āyurveda* herbs can be found in the Resource Material at the end of this book.

A Note about Seasonal and Daily Routines:

It is important to live in accordance with the seasons and Sun. Each season and time of day bring us a combination of the five states of matter described earlier. By understanding the prominence of these elements during the year and day, you can limit any energy excess and dis-ease.

Kapha **season** exists during the coldest parts of winter to the earliest (think mud!) days of spring. Here is how best to balance *kapha* during this time of year:

- Eat warm, dry foods. Early spring growth (dandelion, sprouts, and berries) are best for cleansing that winter sludge.

- Stay active and moving, especially during the early hours of the day (*kapha* time: 6 to 10 a.m.).

- Incorporate activity into your daily routine that moves energy in the body: Neti pot, evening use of nasya (nasal) oil, and tongue scraping.

Pitta **season** exists from the drier stages of spring to the early signs of autumn (just before the leaves dry and fall). Here is how best to balance *pitta* during this time of year:

- Eat cool foods, such as cucumber and zucchini. Use mint and drink aloe juice.

- Limit sun exposure, especially during pitta time (10 to 2 p.m.) Use cooling breath and peppermint essential oil, coconut oil, and aloe to cool down.

- Practice Yin and restorative yoga, Moon bathe, and activate your cooling breath.

Vata **season** exists from the when the leaves dry and fall during autumn to the cold, windy phases of winter. Here is how best to balance vata during this time of year:

- Eat warm, moist, well-cooked foods. Drink plenty of hot tea and cocoa. Chai is an excellent fall tea with lots of warming spices.

- Restorative yoga and meditation are important during this season, as it also coincides with the hectic holidays.

- Incorporate *abhyanga* (self-massage) into your daily routine, using thick, warm sesame oil. Enjoy warm baths.

The Importance of Daily Routines:

Because energy also shifts from *kapha*, *pitta*, and *vata* during the day (think the Sun's movements and placement in the sky), it is important to take part in *dinacharyā* or an *Āyurveda* routine. Use the knowledge you have about energy use and movement for each *dosha*, and act accordingly during each time of day:

- *Kapha* **time:** 6 to 10 a.m. and p.m.
- *Pitta* **time:** 10 to 2 a.m. and p.m.
- *Vata* **time:** 2 to 6 a.m. and p.m.

Here are some tips to maximize your energy (stimulate, transform, or move):

1. Wake early (*kapha* time) to move that energy.

2. Cleanse in the morning: rub hands over face and body to clean aura; wash mouth, eyes, and face; eliminate body waste.

3. Keep oral hygiene a priority throughout the day.

4. Drink water first thing in the morning (warm or room temperature). Add lemon for gut health.

5. Eliminate caffeine.

6. Stick to a regular dietary and exercise schedule. Your body will thank you.

7. Eat according to the *Āyurveda* Clock. Contrary to popular belief, lunch is the most important meal of the day (*pitta* is a hungry energy).

8. Limit stimulation in the evenings, especially blue light and technology.

9. Go to bed before 10 p.m. Create a relaxing pre-bed routine.

10. Enjoy life.

Additional Suggestions:

Here is a list of warm/cool colors, as well as warm/cool aromas and essential oils for use in a diffuser or as perfumes.

Warm Colors: These colors stimulate and intensify. They consist of oranges, reds, yellows, and combinations of those colors. Think Earth tones.

Cool Colors: These colors soothe and relax. They consist of blues, greens, light purple, and combinations of those colors. Think water.

Warm Aromas: These scents are typically associated with fall and winter. Examples include basil, patchouli, frankincense, orange, vanilla, and rose.

Cool Aromas: These scents are typically associated with spring and summer. Examples include jasmine, lavender, sandalwood, mint, and fennel.

Acknowledgements

Although all experiences and people I've met have been a teacher to me, there are a few that I would like to recognize as having a profound impact on how I claimed my path. First, I'd like to thank Sarah Mulvaney for showing me how to heal myself and that my gift of intuition was to be nurtured and not hidden. I would also like to thank Rebecca Damia, who first introduced me to the *Yoga Sūtras* and healing methods through *Āyurveda*, chanting, and self-care. And ultimately, I would like to thank the Source of all, Spirit, for this incredible journey. Without it, this individual consciousness would not enjoy the mystery and devotion that it entails.

Resource Material

Āyurveda

Lad, Vasant. "Food and Nutrition." *The Ayurvedic Institute*, 2020,
www.ayurveda.com/resources/food-and-nutrition.

Lad, Vasant. "Ayurveda: A Brief Introduction and Guide."
The Ayurvedic Institute, 2006,
www.ayurveda.com/resources/articles/ayurveda-a-bri
ef-introduction-and-guide.

Lad, Vasant. "The Daily Routine." *The Ayurvedic Institute*,
2020,
www.ayurveda.com/resources/articles/the-daily-routi
ne.

Lad, Vasant, and Michael Dick. "Doshas: Their Elements
and Attributes." *The Ayurvedic Institute*, 2020,
www.ayurveda.com/resources/articles/doshas-their-el
ements-and-attributes.

Wallis, Tegan. "AYURVEDIC EXERCISE: The Best
Exercise for Your Body Type." *Sukhavati Retreat*,
10 Mar. 2016,
www.sukhavatibali.com/ayurvedic-exercise-the-best
-exercise-for-your-body-type/.

"Your Guide to Ayurvedic Herbs." *The Chopra Center*, 12
Sept. 2018,
chopra.com/your-guide-to-ayurvedic-herbs.

Breathwork (*Prāṇāyāma*)

Knox, Richard. "Harvard Study: Clearing Your Mind Affects Your Genes and Can Lower Your Blood Pressure." *CommonHealth*, WBUR, 6 Apr. 2018, www.wbur.org/commonhealth/2018/04/06/harvard -study-relax-genes.

"Nadi Shodhana Pranayama." Banyan Botanicals, 2020, www.banyanbotanicals.com/info/ayurvedic-living/li ving-ayurveda/yoga/nadi-shodhana-pranayama/.

Novotny, Sarah, and Len Kravitz. "The Science of Breathing." *The University of New Mexico*, www.unm.edu/~lkravitz/Article%20folder/Breathing .html.

Wilson, Kristin. "Breaking Through the Inhale and Exhale Confusion in Yoga." *DOYOU.COM*, 9 Apr. 2015, www.doyou.com/breaking-through-the-inhale-and-e xhale-confusion-in-yoga-42928/.

Meditation (*Saṁyama*)

Gillmore, Lorilee. "Dharana and the Power of Focus." *Banyan Botanicals*, 30 Mar. 2018, www.banyanbotanicals.com/info/blog-the-banyan-in sight/details/dharana-and-the-power-of-focus/.

Postures (*Āsana*)

Bidlake, Erin. "Yoga for Back Care: 6 Directions of the Spine." *Erin Bidlake:* Yoga, *Community Deathcare,* 14 Oct. 2018, erinbidlake.com/yoga-for-back-care-the-six-directions-of-the-spine/?doing_wp_cron=1577554639.4729950428009033203125.

Kaur, Indra. "The Benefits of Asanas Yoga." *The Secretes of* Yoga, 2020, www.thesecretsofyoga.com/yoga-articles/benefits-of-asanas.html.

Savage, Jenny. "Yoga Twists, the Ins and Outs." *Ekhart* Yoga, 19 Apr. 2020, www.ekhartyoga.com/articles/practice/yoga-twists-the-ins-and-outs.

"Seated Yoga Poses: The Health Benefits & 11 Poses to Get You Started." *Liforme,* 2020, liforme.com/blogs/blog/seated-yoga-poses.

Wei, Marlynn. "You Can Do Yoga: A Simple 15-Minute Morning Routine." *Harvard Health Blog,* 21 June 2017, www.health.harvard.edu/blog/you-can-do-yoga-a-simple-15-minute-morning-routine-2017062111921.

Psychology

Ito, T. A., Larsen, J. T., Smith, N. K., & Cacioppo, J. T.
(1998). Negative information weighs more heavily
on the brain: The negativity bias in evaluative
categorizations. *Journal of Personality and Social
Psychology, 75*(4),
887–900. https://doi.org/10.1037/0022-3514.75.4.
887

"Facts & Statistics." *Anxiety and Depression Association of
America, ADAA*, 2018,
adaa.org/about-adaa/press-room/facts-statistics.

Gaspar, Lori. "Yoga Sutra 1.7." *Prairie Yoga*, 7 Feb. 2017,
prairieyoga.org/blog/2017/02/07/yoga-sutra-17.

Sleep (*Nidra*)

"Introduction to Psychology: Stages of Sleep." *Lumen
Learning*,
courses.lumenlearning.com/wsu-sandbox/chapter/s
tages-of-sleep/.

"Sleep Better with Simple Yoga Poses." *Art of Living
(India)*, 2020,

www.artofliving.org/in-en/yoga/health-and-wellness/yoga-for-sleep.

"Sleep Deprivation and Deficiency." *National Heart Lung and Blood Institute*, U.S. Department of Health and Human Services, www.nhlbi.nih.gov/health-topics/sleep-deprivation-and-deficiency.

Wealth and Resources

Depta, Laura. "Global Food Waste and Its Environmental Impact: Green Living." *RESET*, Sept. 2018, en.reset.org/knowledge/global-food-waste-and-its-environmental-impact-09122018.

Sharma, Eesha and Mazar, Nina and Alter, Adam and Ariely, Dan, Financial Deprivation Selectively Shifts Moral Standards and Compromises Moral Decisions (September 10, 2013). Organizational Behavior and Human Decision Processes, September 2013; Rotman School of Management Working Paper No. 2325954. Available at SSRN: https://ssrn.com/abstract=2325954.

"Your Personal Net Worth." *Schwab MoneyWise*, Charles Schwab & Co., Inc., 2020, www.schwabmoneywise.com/public/moneywise/essentials/personal_net_worth.

Yoga

Bachman, Nicolai. *The Path of the* Yoga *Sutras: A Practical Guide to the Core of* Yoga. JAICO Publishing House, 2016.

Corn, Seane. *Revolution of the Soul: Awaken to Love through Raw Truth, Radical Healing, and Conscious Action.* Sounds True, 2019.

Patāñjali. *The Yoga Sūtras of Patāñjali.* Translated by Śrī Svāmī Saccidānanda, Integral Yoga Publications, 2012.

Stern, Eddie. *One Simple Thing: A New Look at the Science of Yoga and How It Can Transform Your Life.* North Point FSG, 2020.

"Yoga and Its Four Parts: Schools of Yoga." *Ajarya Yoga Academy*, 2020, www.ajarya.com/yoga_schools.php.

About the Author

With over 20 years' experience, Melissa Lavery is a writer and editor with work published both online and in print. In 2005, she earned a B.S. in Secondary Education (English and U.S. History) and is a former high school English, journalism, and psychology teacher. In 2012, she earned an M.S. in Psychology (Child and Adolescent Development). Today, she is a stay-at-home parent, virtual assistant, writer, editor, and yoga and *Āyurveda* student. Melissa began her yoga study in 2011 and *Āyurveda* in 2016, since participating in a daily practice that she holds as both sacred and life changing. She continues to channel her education and life experiences into practical guides for helping individuals improve their wellbeing, while making an impact on the collective.

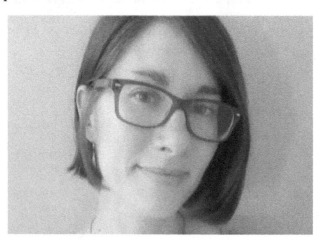